020311

IMMUNOLOGY

A Comprehensive Review

Darla J. Wise and Gordon R. Carter

IMMUNOLOGY
A Comprehensive Review

IOWA STATE UNIVERSITY PRESS

A Blackwell Science Company

DARLA J. WISE is an assistant professor of biology at Concord College in Athens, West Virginia. Dr. Wise has published articles in the areas of immune responses, characterization of enzymes associated with host-pathogen relationships, and DNA-based methods of disease diagnosis. She is associate editor of *Proceedings of the West Virginia Academy of Science*. She has a patent in the area of molecular biology.

GORDON R. CARTER is a professor emeritus at Virginia Polytechnic Institute and State University in Blacksburg, Virginia. His area of expertise is pathogenic microbiology. He has published many scientific papers and is the senior author on more than a dozen textbooks. He has served on the faculties of the University of Toronto and Michigan State University and has served as a consultant on infectious diseases of animals for several international agencies.

© 2002 Iowa State University Press
A Blackwell Science Company
All rights reserved

Iowa State University Press
2121 South State Avenue, Ames, Iowa 50014

Orders: 1-800-862-6657
Office: 1-515-292-0140
Fax: 1-515-292-3348
Web site (secure): www.isupress.com

Authorization to photocopy items for internal or personal use, or the internal or personal use of specific clients, is granted by Iowa State University Press, provided that the base fee of $.10 per copy is paid directly to the Copyright Clearance Center, 222 Rosewood Drive, Danvers, MA 01923. For those organizations that have been granted a photocopy license by CCC, a separate system of payments has been arranged. The fee code for users of the Transactional Reporting Service is 0-8138-1599-1/2002 $.10.

♾ Printed on acid-free paper in the United States of America

First edition, 2002

Library of Congress Cataloging-in-Publication Data

Wise, Darla J.
    Immunology: a comprehensive review / Darla J. Wise and Gordon R. Carter—1st ed.
        p. cm.
    Includes bibliographical references and index.
    ISBN 0-8138-1599-1 (alk. paper)
        1. Immunology [DNLM: 1. Immunity. QW 540 W812i 2001] I. Carter, G. R.
    (Gordon R.) II. Title.
        QR181 .W715 2001
        616.07'9—dc21   2001004465

The last digit is the print number: 9 8 7 6 5 4 3 2 1

Contents

Preface

Saying that immunology is a complex subject is almost an understatement. Most current texts on the subject are large and the sheer mass of technical information presented is frequently intimidating to students. Unlike other subjects, there is little in the way of help—reviews, outlines, and such—for the immunology student.

Our relatively small book was written to aid the immunology student. It presents the essential and basic ideas of immunology in a clear and uncluttered fashion. Although concise, it is comprehensive and a knowledge of its contents will assure the student a high level of understanding of the subject.

Among the book's features are the following:

- Seventeen up-to-date chapters covering all aspects of immunology
- Many figures and tables illustrating principles and summarizing data
- A comprehensive list of milestones in immunology
- A glossary at the end of most chapters as well as a cumulative glossary at the end of the book
- A particularly thorough discussion of immunodiagnostic techniques and AIDS

In conclusion, we think this clear and easy-to-use precis of immunology will greatly aid students in acquiring an acceptable grasp of this difficult and important subject.

Abbreviations
and Greek Letters

ABBREVIATIONS

Ab	antibody
ADCC	antibody dependent cell-mediated immunity
Ag	antigen
AIDS	acquired immune deficiency syndrome
APC	antigen presenting cell
AZT	azidothymidine
BCG	bacille Calmette-Guérin
C	complement
CBH	cutaneous basophil hypersensitivity
CEA	carcino-embryonic antigen
CGD	chronic granulomatous disease
CMI	cell-mediated immunity
CSF	colony-stimulating factor
DTH	delayed-type hypersensitivity
EIA	enzyme-linked immunoassay
ELISA	enzyme-linked immunosorbent assay
Fab	fragment antibody binding
FACS	fluorescent activated cell sorter
FasL	Fas ligand
H	histamine receptor (e.g., H1, H2...)
HIV	human immunodeficiency virus
HLA	human leukocyte antigen
IFN	interferon
Ig	immunoglobulin
IL	interleukin (e.g., IL-1)
GM-SF	granulocyte monocyte stimulating factor
LAK	lymphokinase activated killer cells
LPS	lipopolysaccharide

MAC	membrane attack complex
MCF	macrophage chemotactic factor
MHC	major histocompatibility complex
NK	natural killer cells
PCR	polymerase chain reaction
RAST	radioallergosorbent test
RIA	radioimmunoassay
RTC	reverse transcriptase
SCID	severe combined immunodeficiency (syndrome)
Tc	cytotoxic T cell
TCR	T cell receptor
Td	delayed hypersensitivity T cell
Th	T-helper cell
TNF	tumor necrosis factor
TNFR	tumor necrosis factor receptor
Ts	T-suppressor cell
VSG	variable surface glycoprotein

GREEK LETTERS

α	alpha
β	beta
γ	gamma
δ	delta
μ	mu

IMMUNOLOGY
A Comprehensive Review

CHAPTER 1

Introducing Immunology

The development of the science of immunology, which has burgeoned in the last several decades, is marked by many notable discoveries. Some of the more significant ones are listed at the end of this chapter in the section Milestones in Immunology.

The summary that follows will introduce you to this important and fascinating science.(Terms in boldface are defined in the glossary at the end of the chapter.)

BASIC CONCEPTS

Immunology

Immunology is the science that studies the nature and functioning of the immune system.

Immunity

Immunity is the ability whereby vertebrates protect themselves from infection by microbes, parasites, and other foreign substances that can be referred to as "nonself." This protection is provided by the immune system.

Infection

It seems probable that the main reason for the evolution of the immune system was to protect the body against infection by pathogenic viruses, bacteria, fungi, protozoa, and helminths (parasitic worms).

Immunity to nonself, including the pathogenic agents just mentioned, is divided into natural and acquired components. Acquired immunity is further divided into active (adaptive) and passive immunity.

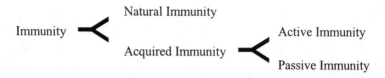

Natural, Native, or Innate Immunity

This is the nonspecific immunity, inborn and unchanging, resulting from the genetic nature of the host; for example, humans are naturally immune to many of the infectious diseases that affect animals. When **antigen** is encountered, these mechanisms always respond in the same manner, regardless of the nature of the antigen.

Natural Resistance

The entry of various microorganisms is prevented by the skin and mucous membranes. By far, the majority of microbes that do gain entry are quickly eliminated by nonspecific defense mechanisms. Those that escape these nonspecific mechanisms can go on to produce infection, at which time specific immune mechanisms (the immune response) will be directed against them.

Active Immunity/Adaptive Immunity

This is the immunity or protection that results from development of the immune response when an individual is stimulated by an antigen such as those associated with invading microorganisms. This response is specific to a particular antigen. If presented with a new antigen, the response will not be the same as a response to another antigen.

Passive Immunity

This is immunity received by a nonimmune individual from an immune individual. An example is the injection of a human with tetanus anti-toxin (immunity) produced in horses to protect against tetanus.

Immune System

This complex system comprises all the cells and molecules that protect against invading organisms and foreign substances, including tumors.

Immune Response

This is the specific response to antigen and includes humoral immunity and cell-mediated immunity.

The immune system of vertebrates has evolved two principal strategies for defending the body against the intrusion of disease agents and other foreign substances. They are cell-mediated immunity (cellular immunity) and humoral immunity (mediated by **antibodies**). Their roles in protecting the host are outlined in figure 1.1.

Cell-Mediated Immunity (CMI)/Cellular Immunity

A form of acquired immunity that is dependent on the action of various types of **T lymphocytes.** This form of immunity can be transferred passively with "immune cells" but not with **immune serum.**

Cell-mediated immunity is particularly important in defending against intracellular microbes such as *Salmonella, Listeria,* and the causes of tuberculosis and the typhus fevers.

Humoral Immunity

A form of acquired immunity mediated by specific antibodies occurring in the blood and tissue fluids of the body. These antibodies, and thus protection, can be transferred to a nonimmune individual by immune sera (passive immunization). The interaction between humoral and cell-mediated responses determines the overall immune response.

Some important features of the acquired immune response as they relate to infection and various defense mechanisms are summarized in figure 1.2.

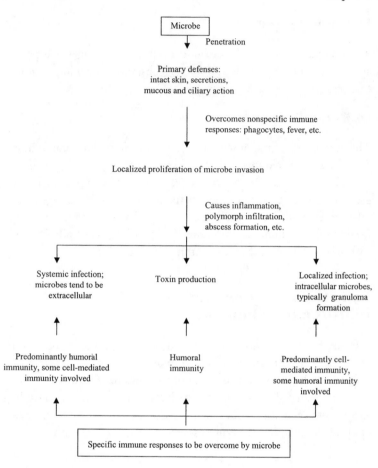

Figure 1.1. Host-pathogen interactions in the production of disease. Note that a pathogen must evade both the natural and specific immune responses of the host in order to achieve infection. The pathogens possess a variety of mechanisms by which they attempt to circumvent the immune responses of the host.

The scope of immunology is broad. Several of the many areas of practical importance are immunity to various disease agents, allergy/hypersensitivity, autoimmune diseases, immunotherapy, tumor immunology, transplant, graft rejection, vaccination, and immunodiagnostic techniques.

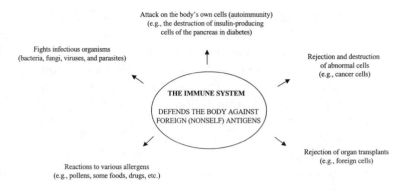

Figure 1.2. Principal activities of the immune system in defense of the body

MILESTONES IN IMMUNOLOGY

1700s (early) Variolation was introduced from the Middle East to Western countries. It consisted of applying smallpox scabs to skin scratches. It was effective in preventing smallpox.

1796 Edward Jenner employed cowpox virus to vaccinate humans against smallpox. The difference between the two viruses is now known to be about a dozen genes.

1879 Louis Pasteur developed a live attenuated vaccine to prevent fowl cholera, an important bacterial disease of domestic and wild fowl.

1882 Eli Metchnikoff is credited with the discovery of phagocytes and he strongly contended that they were important in resistance to infectious disease.

1885 Pasteur developed an effective rabies vaccine. Initially this vaccine consisted of a suspension of dried spinal cord of a rabbit that had been infected with virulent rabies virus.

1890 In Robert Koch's laboratory, Emil von Bering and Shabasaburu Kitasato discovered tetanus toxin and prepared tetanus antitoxin (antibody to tetanus toxin) in rabbits. In the same laboratory diphtheria toxin was identified, antitoxin produced, and successful passive immunization begun.

1893–1895 The combined observations of Buchner, Pfeiffer, and Bordet led to the recognition of complement and antibodies.

1900 Karl Landsteiner identified the human A, B, and O blood groups.

The precipitin test was used by Nuttall, Wassermann, and Schutze to distinguish between the milk of humans, cows, and goats. Paul Ehrlich, who is considered the father of immunochemistry, made many contributions to the science of immunology including the first selective theory termed the "side-chain theory." It has been supplanted by the clonal selection theory of Sir MacFarlane Burnet. Ehrlich's concept of *horror autotoxicus* that immunity to self could have damaging consequences was a founding principle of immunology.

1900s Vaccines were introduced for the prevention of typhoid and cholera.

1902 Portier and Richet demonstrated anaphylaxis.

1903 Arthus demonstrated what is now called the Arthus reaction.

1905 von Pirquet and Schick elucidated the cause of serum sickness.

1914–1918 Passive serum treatment was used extensively in the First World War to prevent tetanus and gas gangrene.

1916–1933 Cooke made an extensive study of immediate type sensitivity to pollen extracts that contributed greatly to the understanding of allergy.

1920s BCG (Bacille Calmette-Guérin), a live vaccine, was developed for the prevention of tuberculosis.

1921 Prausnitz and Kustner showed that the active agent of immediate hypersensitivity circulates in the blood. This laid the groundwork for the study of allergies.

1923 Glenny and Ramon independently discovered that formaldehyde treatment of several toxins destroyed their toxicity but not their immunogenicity. These attenuated toxins are known as toxoids and they have been widely used to prevent several important bacterial diseases, including tetanus, diphtheria, and botulism.

1930s Diphtheria and yellow fever vaccines were introduced.

1932 Rich and Lewis studying the reaction to tuberculin laid the groundwork for the later identification of the migration inhibitory factor.

1940s Chase showed that antigen-specific delayed-type hypersensitivity could be transferred using lymphocytes from the hypersensitive animal. These observations lead to the eventual recognition of the second arm of the immune response, cell-mediated immunity.
Influenza and whooping cough vaccines were introduced.

1943 Medawar, through a series of skin-grafting experiments in rabbits, showed that graft rejection was immunological in nature.

1945 Owen found that genetically distinct twin calves (fraternal twins) called freemartin twins are completely tolerant of each other's blood although genetically different. The principle was established that anything we are exposed to prior to birth will be regarded as self (immunological tolerance).

1950 Glick and Chang discovered the important role of the bursa of Fabricius in the production of antibodies.

1950s Burnet with associates developed over a number of years the clonal selection theory of antibody production.

1952 Brunton provided the first medical report linking a clinical disease (Brunton's agammaglobulinemia) with an immune defect.

1955–1959 The clonal selection theory was proposed and developed by Niels Jerne, David Talmage, and MacFarlane Burnet.

1955–1960 Salk introduced a killed virus poliomyelitis vaccine. Sabin developed an attenuated oral vaccine. Both vaccines were effective and are still widely used.

1956 Rose and Witebsky showed that their experimental thyroiditis in rabbits was an autoimmune disease and that the damage to the thyroid was the same as that seen in human Hashimoto's thyroiditis. The latter was confirmed as an autoimmune disease.

1960s The discovery of T cells; Measles and rubella vaccines were introduced.

1961–1962 Jaques Miller discovered the role of the thymus in cellular immunity.

Noel Warner et al. described the humoral immune and cellular immune responses as independent entities.

1964–1968 Elucidation of the T and B cell interactions in the generation of the immune response.

1965 DiGeorge found that athymic infants were immunodeficient (e.g., didn't reject grafts) and this led to elucidation of the role of the thymus. It was concluded from this and from the observations of Good and others that the immune system consisted of two separate arms, the humoral or antibody-mediated response and the cell-mediated immune response.

1966 The early work of Rich and Lewis (1932) was extended by two research groups leading to the identification of the migration inhibitory factor (MIF). This factor was the first lymphokine (cytokine) identified and it started a search for additional cytokines by many researchers over several years.

1970s Borel and associates discovered the now widely used immunosuppressive compound, cyclosporin A.

1974 Zinkernagel and Doherty described major histocompatibility complex (MHC) restriction.

1975 Miltsein and Kohler successfully produced monoclonal antibodies.

1982 Introduction of recombinant hepatitis B vaccine made in yeast cells.

1984 Robert Good attempted to treat severe combined immunodeficiency (SCID) by bone marrow transplant; it ultimately failed.

1985 Immunoglobulin genes were identified by Tonegawa et al.

1985–1987 T cell receptor genes were identified by Leroy Hood et al.

1987 Bjorkman determined the structure of the major histocompatibility complex class I molecule.

1990 Molecular differences between the genes for blood groups were described by Yamamoto et al.

The National Institutes of Health (NIH) used gene therapy to treat SCID *in vitro* utilizing cultured T cells.

1985–1997+ Development of techniques to quickly identify different facets of the immune system, such as immune cells, antibodies, and cytokines.

GLOSSARY

Antibody—a glycoprotein, one of five classes of immunoglobulins, produced by **plasma cells.** It has the capacity to recognize and bind to foreign molecules such as those on the surface of pathogenic organisms.

Antigen—a substance, usually external to the body but occasionally within the body, which the immune system recognizes as foreign or nonself. When thus recognized, it can elicit a specific antibody that reacts with it.

Immune sera—sera that contain protective antibodies.

Plasma cells—mature B cells that have been stimulated by the combination of specific antigen and cytokines (intercellular mediators) to produce antibodies.

T lymphocytes—cells of the immune system that mature in the thymus and are involved in the cell-mediated immune response.

CHAPTER 2

The Hemopoietic and Lymphopoietic Cells

The immune system consists of a complex network of different cells and their products that interact in the immune response. The function of the immune response is to provide resistance to substances often described as "nonself."

The components comprising the immune system arise in the fetal bone marrow between the third and sixth month of fetal life. Cells called stem cells arise and multiply in the bone marrow to yield two major cell lines, the hemopoietic (*poiesis* = producing) cells and the lymphopoietic cells. These stem cells are pleuripotent, that is, many different cell types arise from the same progenitor cell based upon the microenvironment of **cytokines** and other factors present during differentiation.

In the process of hemopoiesis, the precursor hemopoietic cells give rise to red blood cells (erythrocytes) and white blood cells. Red blood cells have no role in the immune system. In the process of lymphopoiesis, lymphocytes develop from precursor lymphopoietic cells.

THE HEMOPOIETIC SYSTEM

Stem cells give rise to hemopoietic stem cells, which give rise to the following cell types:

Megakaryocyte. This cell gives rise to **platelets** (thrombocytes), which are involved in blood clotting and inflammation.

Erythroid stem cells. These differentiate into red blood cells.

Granulocyte-monocyte precursor cells. These differentiate into various cells of the myeloid series (granular leukocytes and mononuclear

13

phagocytes). Differentiation is dependent on various growth or colony stimulating factors.

The four cell types listed below are referred to as granulocytes:

Basophil. This cell contains large basophilic granules that contain **heparin** and **vasoactive amines,** which are important in inflammation. Basophils constitute up to 1 percent of circulating leukocytes; their numbers increase during inflammation.

Mast cell. This large tissue cell, which is thought to originate from the bone marrow, resembles closely the basophil in appearance and function. The basophilic granules that it contains are similar but smaller than those of the basophil. Two **phenotypically** different populations of mast cells have been described, mucosal mast cells and connective tissue mast cells.

Neutrophil (polymorph). This very common leukocyte is a short-lived phagocytic cell with granules that contain a number of bactericidal compounds. Neutrophils, frequently called polymorphonuclear leukocytes, are the most numerous of the circulating leukocytes constituting approximately 60 to 70 percent in humans. Microscopically they have an irregularly shaped, multilobed nucleus.

Eosinophil. This leukocyte has large granules containing a number of proteins that are injurious to parasites including **helminths.** Eosinophils stain readily with the acidic dye eosin and have a bilobed nucleus. Under normal circumstances, they comprise up to 5 percent of circulating leukocytes.

Colony-stimulating factors (CFS). Although not cells, these factors are produced by various cells and are important in the differentiation of granulocytes and monocytes. Some of the CSFs are available in pure form as a result of genetic engineering. Each has been shown to have multiple effects.

The granulocyte-monocyte common precursor also gives rise to:

Monocytes. These are large nucleated phagocytic cells found in the blood. When they migrate into tissues and organs they are referred to as macrophages.

Macrophage. This is the main phagocyte of tissues, organs and such serous membranes as the pleura and peritoneum.

THE LYMPHOPOIETIC SYSTEM

Stem cells give rise to lymphopoietic stem cells, which are presumed to differentiate into T and B lymphocytes after processing in the thymus and bursa equivalent (bursa, bone marrow, or fetal liver), respectively (fig. 2.1).

The thymus is a two-lobed organ about the size of a walnut located above the heart. After the age of sixteen the thymus begins a progressive deterioration. The pre-T cells are processed in the thymus to develop into T lymphocytes. Small **peptides,** such as the thymic hormone, thymosin, are thought to assist in the differentiation of T lymphocytes. A summary of the major features of lymphopoietic cells is provided in table 2.1.

T lymphocytes (T for thymus; also called T cells). They comprise about 75 percent of lymphocytes in the blood, are responsible for cell-mediated immunity, and do not produce antibodies. They have different receptor sites than B lymphocytes. T cells can be subdivided into T-cytotoxic (Tc) and T-helper (Th) cells based upon cell surface markers and cell function.

Bursa of Fabricius. A lymphoid organ located near the **cloacal opening** of the bird. It processes lymphoid stem cells to produce B (for bursa) lymphocytes (also called B cells). Humans do not have a bursa and it is thought that the bursa equivalents in humans are the bone marrow and the fetal liver.

B lymphocytes (B for bursa; also called B cells). Most B cells migrate from the bone marrow and liver to secondary lymphoid organs and tissues throughout the body. Roughly 20 percent remain in the circulation.

Plasma cells. B lymphocytes can transform into plasma cells, which produce antibodies and thus are responsible for humoral immunity. Plasma cells are found mainly in the spleen and lymphoid tissue and only rarely in the blood; however, the antibodies readily enter the circulation.

Natural killer cell (NK cell). These cytotoxic lymphocytes, which comprise approximately 5 to 15 percent of circulating lymphocytes, lack the phenotypic markers of T and B cells. They are morphologically distinguishable from T cells and have the capacity to kill certain tumor cells and virus-infected cells. The mechanism used for antigen recognition is the lack of **major histocompatibility complex**

(**MHC**) markers on cell surfaces and their mechanism of killing is similar to that of cytotoxic T cells.

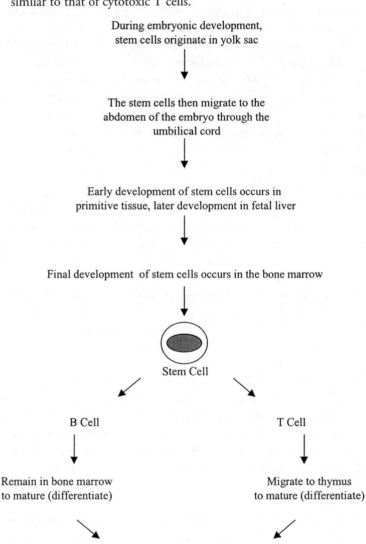

Figure 2.1. Ontogeny of T cells and B cells

Table 2.1. Major Features of Lymphopoietic Cells

Features	T cells	B cells	NK cells	Monocytes and macrophages
Presentation of antigen	no	yes	no	yes
Recognition of antigen	yes	yes	no	no
Production of antibody	no	yes	no	no
Cellular immunity	yes	no	yes	yes
Capable of phagocytosis	no	no	no	yes
Cytotoxicity	yes	no	yes	yes

LYMPHOID ORGANS

The primary lymphoid organs serve as the sites of maturation for lymphocytes, and include the bone marrow and the thymus.

The secondary lymphoid organs, the spleen and lymph nodes, are responsible for lymphocyte interaction with antigen, other immune cells, and accessory cells. The lymph nodes are located strategically throughout the body. In addition, tonsils, adenoids, the vermiform appendix, and Peyer's patches of the ileum region of the small intestine all consist of lymphoid tissue. Clusters of lymphoid tissue, like the Peyer's patches, are also found in mucous and other membranes and throughout various tissues.

THE LYMPHATIC SYSTEM

Blood reaches all tissues via capillaries. The fluid component of the blood seeps out of the capillaries carrying food and oxygen into tissues. It picks up carbon dioxide and other metabolic waste products and what is now referred to as lymph returns to the heart via the lymphatic system (also known as the second circulatory system). The lymphatic system consists of a blindly terminating meshwork of lymph capillaries or lacteals. Unlike blood capillaries, lymph vessels do not have nonreturn valves. The returning lymph flows from the lacteals into larger, then larger lymph vessels—all the time passing through lymph nodes. The fluid then enters the large thoracic duct, the venous system, and finally the heart.

The lymph nodes, as mentioned earlier, are placed strategically (e.g., the groin, armpit, and chest) along the return route of the lymph. The lymph nodes "examine" the returning lymph for foreign matter. Exogenous (from outside) matter, frequently microorganisms, triggers a defensive immune response. This filtering system is remarkably efficient in that it examines the returning lymph from literally every cubic centimeter of the body.

GLOSSARY

Cloacal opening—the common chamber of avian species into which the intestine and urinary tracts open and discharge wastes.

Cytokines—soluble molecules that mediate interactions between cells.

Helminths—parasitic worms.

Heparin—a compound, which occurs in the liver and lungs, that is used to prolong the clotting time of blood.

Major histocompatibility complex (MHC)—the collection of genes coding for the self-marking proteins or major histocompatibility antigens. These antigens occur on the surface of all body cells and identify them as belonging to the body and not foreign. Some MHC antigens appear on the surface of cells of the immune system. The human MHC region is known as the HLA (human leukocyte antigen) region and is located on chromosome 6.

Peptide—a compound consisting of two or several amino acids.

Phenotype—the expressed character of an organism.

Platelet—a small nonnucleated disc found in mammalian blood that is important in blood clotting.

Vasoactive amines—compounds produced by various cells that act on endothelium (lining cells of blood vessels) and smooth muscle of the local vasculature.

CHAPTER 3

Natural Immunity and Resistance

As stated in chapter 1, immunity or resistance to foreign substances (nonself), including microorganisms, is divided into natural immunity and acquired immunity (adaptive immunity). The mechanisms of natural immunity operate in conjunction with the mechanisms of adaptive immunity. Innate or native immunity encompasses an organism's ability to defend itself from assaults generated by its environment. The main features of natural immunity and resistance are summarized below. Although discussed by categories, it should be kept in mind that the different mechanisms may act simultaneously.

NATURAL OR NATIVE IMMUNITY

This is the nonspecific immunity attributed to the genetic makeup of the individual, such as the immunity of humans to many infectious diseases that affect animals. These mechanisms occur in precisely the same manner, regardless of the nature of the antigen. For example, phagocytes will engulf and destroy any foreign invader in exactly the same manner, whether it is a bacterium or virus.

PHYSICAL AND CHEMICAL BARRIERS

The major physical barrier of vertebrates against the onslaught of various microorganisms is the skin. As long as the integrity of the skin is intact, most microorganisms and other substances cannot readily penetrate this barrier. Some microorganisms may attempt to bypass the barrier of the skin by gaining access via the sebaceous glands and hair follicles. However, this is discouraged chemically by the acid pH of sweat and sebaceous secretions and associated fatty acids and enzymes, such as

19

lysozyme. The combinations of these chemical factors provide an antimicrobial barrier against potential penetration of the intact skin.

If the skin is intact, the next most obvious port of entry for a microbe is via the respiratory, alimentary, or urogenital tracts. To deter this, the surfaces of these tracts are lined with ciliated epithelial cells covered with a layer of mucus. The ciliated cells maintain a constant movement of the mucus toward the outside of the body. The mucus effectively traps any potential microbes and the action of the cilia moves the invader back out into the environment. The physical action of the cilia is often coupled with the chemical activity of enzymes, such as the hydrolytic enzymes of saliva, or decreased pH as in the stomach and vagina. In addition, below the epithelial barrier are many macrophages, which are available to phagocytize and destroy microbes that may penetrate this barrier.

INFLAMMATION

This is the localized tissue reaction to injury caused by physical and chemical agents, and by introduction of foreign substances to tissues, including microorganisms. Inflammation is characterized by redness, pain, heat, and swelling. The functions of inflammation are (1) to destroy and remove a deleterious agent, if possible; (2) if it cannot be removed, to sequester the injury to a localized area within the body; and (3) to repair any damage that may have resulted from the injury.

Three stages characterize the inflammatory response:

1. **Vasodilation** at the site of injury causes the redness and heat associated with inflammation, and the increased capillary permeability allows soluble mediators to reach the site. This fluid movement into the tissue causes the swelling (edema) associated with inflammation. Pain is the result of nerve damage, inflammation, and the pressure of edema associated with the presence of toxins.

   Histamine, kinins, prostaglandins, and leukotrienes are released by or in response to damaged cells. Phagocytic granulocytes, platelets, mast cells, and basophils release additional histamine at the site of injury. The kinins stimulate vasodilation and increase the permeability of blood vessels. Kinins are present in the blood plasma and once activated, stimulate chemotaxis of phagocytes, particularly neutrophils, to the site. The prostaglandins enhance the activity of both histamine and the kinins, aiding in the emigration of phagocytes. Leukotrienes are produced by mast cells and basophils and act to increase capillary permeability and increase phagocytosis. Platelets also aid in clot formation at the site, and thus sequester the site.

2. Migration of leukocytes into the site, particularly the phagocytes (neutrophils and macrophages) that are needed to destroy and remove pathogens and damaged tissue cells. They typically appear within an hour after tissue damage or bacterial infiltration. Phagocytes move from the bloodstream by **margination** and **emigration**. Neutrophils are typically first on the scene, followed by the monocytes (in the process maturing into macrophages).

3. Tissue repair. This is the process whereby dead or damaged cells are replaced. It begins during the earlier stages of the inflammatory response but cannot be completed unless all harmful products have been neutralized or removed from the site. Ability to repair tissue is dependent upon the amount of damage and tissue type.

Chemotaxis, with reference to inflammation, denotes the movement of cells, for instance leukocytes, to the site of injury in response to various chemicals referred to as chemotactic factors.

C5a, a fragment of one of the **complement** components attracts neutrophils and macrophages to the site of inflammation and enables them to adhere to endothelial cells of capillaries.

C3a and C5a, complement pathway fragments, are referred to as anaphylatoxins; they induce the degranulation of mast cells and basophils. This degranulation includes the release of histamine, which increases capillary permeability and smooth muscle contraction leading to a local edema.

FEVER

Fever is the systemic response to injury, most frequently caused by endotoxins or viruses. Body temperature is regulated by the hypothalamus. Phagocytosis and destruction of gram-negative bacteria by phagocytes allow for the release of the bacterial **lipopolysaccharide** (LPS). In response to the presence of the LPS, the phagocytes secrete **interleukin-1** (IL-1). The presence of IL-1 in the bloodstream is detected by the hypothalamus, which responds by secreting **prostaglandins**. The prostaglandin levels then stimulate the hypothalamus to increase body temperature. To aid in this elevation of temperature, the body responds by constricting blood vessels, increasing the rate of metabolism, and shivering ("chills"). The body will maintain this elevated temperature until IL-1 is no longer present. Fever is thought to aid in the immune response in the following ways: First, IL-1 helps stimulate T lymphocytes. Second, interferons (see section below) have increased activity at higher temperatures. Third, the increased temperature speeds up the body's repair mechanisms.

PHAGOCYTOSIS

This is the "eating" or engulfment of a foreign substance, particle, or microorganism by phagocytes (mainly macrophages and neutrophils). Most of the foreign material gaining entrance to skin and mucous membranes is disposed of by phagocytosis.

The sequence of the main events in phagocytosis is attachment, endocytosis (ingestion or engulfment), and digestion. It is necessary that phagocytes recognize the foreign material, that is, the invading microorganism. Phagocytes have **receptors** on their surface that attach nonspecifically to many different microorganisms. The component of complement, C3b, is often found on the surface of many microbes as the result of activating the alternate pathway of complement (see chapter 5). Phagocytes have receptors for the complement protein, C3b, which enhances attachment; this is called **opsonization**. The importance of opsonization is illustrated by the fact that a deficiency of C3 in individuals leads to recurrence of bacterial infections.

Phagocytes engulf foreign material and microorganisms by extending **pseudopodia** around them and thus internalizing them in what is termed a phagosome (an intracellular vesicle).

Lysosomes are "packages" of hydrolytic enzymes found in phagocytic cells. Once a phagosome and a lysosome fuse, the enzymes digest the material in phagosomes. There are also vesicles in phagocytic cells that contain lysozyme and other enzymes that act against phagocytized material. Lysozyme (muramidase) produced by phagocytes attacks the cell wall of gram-positive bacteria. It also potentiates the action of complement against gram-negative bacteria. The granules found in the cells called granulocytes, namely, neutrophils, basophils, and eosinophils, also contain the various enzymes just mentioned.

Phagocytes, by various biochemical reactions, produce toxic forms of oxygen, such as hydrogen peroxide, superoxide, and hydroxyl radicals, which aid in killing ingested bacteria.

EXTRACELLULAR KILLING

This involves the killing of some tumor or virus-infected cells that are recognized by natural killer (NK) cells. In this killing process, target cells are destroyed by the release of granules from NK cells containing a variety of substances, such as perforins, which form **transmembrane** pores in the target cell. Other molecules, such as granzymes, stimulate **apoptosis** within the target cell.

Interferons are also involved in nonspecific natural resistance.

INTERFERONS

These comprise three different proteins designated alpha, beta, and gamma. All have a nonspecific action against viruses, but alpha and beta are the more potent. Alpha interferon comprises several variant proteins. The alpha and beta interferons, which are produced by monocytes, bind to an individual's cells and inhibit viral replication within them. Interferons also work by decreasing the availability of iron to microbes. Excess iron suppresses chemotaxis and phagocytosis by immune cells.

NATURAL KILLER (NK) CELLS

These are large cytotoxic lymphocytes containing cytoplasmic granules. They are able to kill cells infected with viruses, and certain sensitive tumor cells. The mechanism of killing is similar to that of cytotoxic T lymphocytes. NK cells have granules containing granzymes, a family of serine **proteases**, which have a role in lymphocyte-mediated cytotoxicity.

GLOSSARY

Apoptosis—a form of programmed cell death characterized by the fragmentation of nuclear DNA.

Complement—a complex of serum proteins that act with and without specific antibody in a number of processes including inflammation, activation of phagocytosis, and lytic action on cell membranes.

Emigration—movement between endothelial cells and into the tissue at the site of injury.

Interleukins (IL)—a number of low-molecular-weight proteins produced by lymphocytes and monocytes that mainly function in the regulation of the immune system.

Lipopolysaccharides—these have a lipid linked to a polysaccharide. They are derived from gram-negative bacteria and have various functions including adjuvancy (enhances the immune response) and acting as a mitogen for B cells.

Lysozyme—an enzyme found in saliva, tears, and nasal secretions that mainly lyses gram-positive bacteria.

Margination—sticking to the endothelium.

Opsonization—the promotion of phagocytosis by specific antibody in conjunction with complement.

Prostaglandins—a number of hormonelike compounds that have a variety of functions as inflammatory mediators.

Protease—an enzyme that hydrolyzes or breaks down protein.

Pseudopodium—the temporary protrusion or retractile process of the protoplasm of a cell.

Receptor—a cell surface molecule that binds particular proteins or peptides.

Transmembrane—across or through the cell membrane.

Vasodilation—widening of the lumen of blood vessels resulting in increased blood supply.

CHAPTER 4

The Nature of Antigens

Substances that interact with the immune system and elicit an immune response are either immunogens or antigens. Any substance that is capable of stimulating an immune response is referred to as an immunogen. In contrast, those substances that are capable of stimulating specific immune responses by binding with specific lymphocytes or antibodies are referred to as antigens. Simply stated, all antigens are immunogens but not all immunogens are antigens. This chapter will primarily focus on antigens. When antigens are recognized as foreign by the immune system, the specific immune response elicited may involve antibody production (humoral immunity) and/or cell-mediated immunity.

The features of an antigen that make it immunogenic include foreignness, high molecular weight, and chemical complexity. Other features such as susceptibility of the antigen to enzymatic **catabolism** and the genetic background of the individual (major histocompatibility complex molecules, T cell and B cell repertoires, etc.) may also have roles in the immunogenicity of an antigen.

As will be discussed in greater detail in chapters 7 and 8, those T and B cells responding to self antigens are deleted or anergized (**anergy**) so that the individual does not typically respond to self antigens. However, contact with a substance that is very different from self antigens is recognized as nonself and will therefore trigger an immune response. In general, the more foreign a substance, the more immunogenic. The exceptions to this rule are those individuals that recognize self antigens as foreign. This results in immune responses mounted against self tissue and is referred to as **autoimmunity** (see chapter 12).

A wide variety of macromolecules that are foreign to the individual can act as antigens. In molecular weight they are fairly high (>6000 **daltons**) and include almost all proteins, lipoproteins, peptides, glycoproteins, many polysaccharides, some nucleic acids, and techoic acids (polymers from bacteria). The larger and more chemically complex the antigen molecule the stronger the immune response. Typically, small substances (<1000 daltons) are not immunogenic. In the range 1000 to 6000 daltons, substances may or may not be immunogenic, depending upon other features of the substance. Those that are large (>6000 daltons) are usually immunogenic.

Another aspect of immunogenicity is chemical complexity. Some antigens are of sufficient molecular weight (>6000 daltons), but still fail to be immunogenic due to a lack of chemical complexity. For example, the capsule of *Bacillus anthracis*, a bacterium that causes anthrax, consists of a **homopolymer** of poly-gamma-D-glutamic acid that is approximately 50,000 daltons. Due to the lack of chemical complexity of the capsule, it is not immunogenic and therefore does not stimulate an immune response.

In some respects, susceptibility to enzymatic degradation is a double-edged sword that applies primarily to protein antigens. If a particular protein cannot be enzymatically degraded, it cannot undergo processing by **antigen presenting cells**. As a direct result, this antigen will not be presented to T cells and therefore will not stimulate an immune response. Alternatively, if a protein is easily degraded into its constituent amino acids before processing and presentation can occur, the probability of the **epitope** being presented to specific T cells is small. This will again result in no specific T cell stimulation to the particular protein.

Last, there is a genetic component associated with the immunogenicity of an antigen. The major histocompatibility complex (MHC) molecules, which are inherited, are capable of binding only to particular amino acid sequences. In this manner, they "select" which epitopes of the processed antigen will be presented to T cells. Also, the particular T and B cells present in an individual at a given time will determine whether or not the proper T and/or B cells necessary to respond to a specific antigen are present.

HAPTENS

Haptens are low-molecular-weight (<1000 daltons) substances that can combine with specific antibody molecules, but by themselves are not able to initiate antibody formation. They are individual antigenic determinants and can include amino acids, sugars, and small polymers. When haptens are chemically bound to a carrier molecule, such as a protein, they may induce a specific antibody response. This chemical binding of a hapten and carrier molecule sometimes takes place *in vivo*, commonly when the hapten combines with cell-surface proteins or circulating-blood proteins. A good example of how some low-molecular-weight drugs can induce an immune response is the case of the antibiotic chloramphenicol (approximately 323 daltons). The initial exposure of an individual to chloramphenicol results in the chloramphenicol binding to cell-surface proteins on white blood cells. As a result these antigens may now be recognized as foreign and elicit a humoral immune response, and the white cells become a target for complement-mediated lysis or phagocytosis. The clinical result of this is agranulocytosis, a decrease in the number of white cells with mainly neutrophils destroyed.

B LYMPHOCYTES

Some important properties of B lymphocytes (B cells) are summarized in table 4.1. B cells, when stimulated by specific antigen, are transformed into plasma cells that secrete antibodies into the blood stream. For a detailed description of this process see chapter 7.

Macromolecular antigens have on their surface small epitopes (antigenic determinants) that can be recognized by specific antibody. The specific immune response recognizes and reacts with only a small part of the antigen molecule. A protein antigen with a molecular weight of 15,000 daltons, consisting of about 125 amino acids, will have an antigenic determinant consisting of about 7 to 22 amino-acid sequences. Substitution of one amino acid for another in the antigenic determinant changes the shape of the determinant and its specificity. With 20 different amino acids, an enormous number of combinations of 7 amino acids are possible. Antigenic determinants include substances such as amino acid side chains, sugars, aromatic groups, organic acids and bases, and hydrocarbons.

Antibodies are formed most readily to epitopes that are on the surface of the foreign macromolecule or to terminal residues, such as sugars of a polymer chain. A cell or virus possesses a mosaic of antigens, including various proteins and polysaccharides, all of which are potential antigens.

Table 4.1. Selected Properties of B and T Lymphocytes

Property	B lymphocytes	T lymphocytes
Origin	Bone marrow	Bone marrow
Sites of maturation	Bone marrow	Thymus
Longevity of cells	Days to years	Months to years
Surface antigens present	Immunoglobulin Complement receptors MHC class II molecules	T cell receptor CD4 or CD8
Type of antigen recognized	Recognition of proteins, carbohydrates, nucleic acids, and lipids; all usually in native state	Processed protein antigens complexed with either MHC class I or class II molecules
Response to antigen	Specific; proliferation and differentiation into plasma cells and memory cells	Specific; proliferation and secretion of cytokines
Roles in the immune response	Production of antibodies, antigen presenting cell for T cells	Production of cytokines; Delayed-type hypersensitivity; Mediate immune response: Humoral vs CMI; Cytotoxicity suppression of immune responses

As will be pointed out later in the discussion of the immune response, the antibody response is remarkably specific; distinguishing between compounds as closely related as glucose and galactose, differing in a hydroxyl group. However, the specificity is not absolute. A homologous antigen is one that only interacts with the antibody it induced; other antigens that react with the same antibody are called heterologous antigens. The interaction that occurs between an antibody and a heterologous antigen is referred to as a cross-reaction. Such reactions are important in immunodiagnostics.

T LYMPHOCYTES

Some important properties of T lymphocytes (T cells) are summarized in table 4.1.

T cells that are involved in the cell-mediated response only recognize peptides derived from processed protein antigens (see below). The T cell receptors only interact with the processed protein antigenic determinant in the context of the MHC molecule and not with the antigen molecule as a whole. The processed antigens, the peptides resulting from the enzymatic degradation of the antigen, are presented to T cells on the surface of antigen-presenting cells complexed with MHC molecules. In contrast to the conformational determinants recognized by antibodies, the epitopes for T cells usually consist of linear portions of protein eight to fifteen amino acids in length. Antigen processing and presentation are therefore restricted to short peptides of protein antigens with primary protein structure. Higher levels of protein structure (secondary, tertiary, and quaternary) are not a factor in the cell-mediated immune response.

T cells can basically be broken down into two subgroups. Those that bear the CD4 marker are known as T-helper (Th) cells and respond to antigen complexed with the MHC class II molecule. Those T cells that bear the CD8 surface marker are T-cytotoxic (Tc) cells and respond to antigen complexed with the MHC class I molecule.

ANTIGEN PROCESSING

Protein antigens are degraded to form small peptides that bind to major histocompatibility complex (MHC) molecules so they can be presented to the T cell receptor.

The pathways of antigen processing are different depending on the class of the MHC antigens. The class I MHC antigens bind to peptides from intracellular sources, whereas class II MHC antigens bind to peptides from extracellular sources. This is important in that some pathogenic microorganisms are predominantly intracellular parasites whereas others are mainly extracellular pathogens. Additional information and illustrations on this subject are presented in chapter 6 under the subheading Antigen Processing and Presentation.

GLOSSARY

Anergy—the phenomenon whereby lymphocytes that have been primed by an antigen fail to respond on second contact with the antigen.

Antigen presenting cell—a cell capable of breaking down protein antigens and eventually displaying the peptide fragments complexed with the major histocompatibility complex on the surface of the cell. Once on the cell surface, the antigen peptide fragment plus major histocompatibility complex are available to intereact with specific T cells. Some examples of antigen presenting cells include macrophages, Langerhans cells, dendritic cells, and B cells.

Autoimmunity—the production of antibody-mediated or cell-mediated immunity to the constituents of the body's own tissues.

Catabolism—the breakdown of inorganic or organic compounds, usually leading to the production of energy.

Dalton—a unit of mass used to express masses of atoms, molecules, and nuclear particles. It is equal to one-twelfth of the weight of the carbon 12 atom; it is also called an atomic mass unit.

Epitope—an antigenic determinant. It stimulates an immune response and binds specifically to antibody.

Homopolymer—a polymer consisting of identical monomer (one that can undergo polymerization) units.

Immunological tolerance—a state of nonreactivity to antigen that ordinarily would induce humoral or cell-mediated immunity. Immune tolerance may be produced in adults from administration of large or small amounts of antigen or contact with antigen in fetal or early postnatal life.

CHAPTER 5

The Complement System

The complement system consists of at least twenty serum proteins that interact in a complex reaction sequence referred to as the complement cascade. The manifestations of these interactions are inflammation, phagocytosis, and lysis of foreign cells. The proteins of the system are referred to collectively as complement because their action complements certain antibody-mediated reactions.

The complement system employs two pathways to achieve its ends: the classical and the alternative pathways. Proteins of the complement system (CS) make up about 5 percent of the serum protein of vertebrates. The proteins of the classical pathway are designated by numbers (following C for complement) ranging from C1 through C9.

The alternate pathway comprises proteins called factor B and factor D along with C3 and C5 through C9 proteins of the classical pathway. Both pathways are discussed below.

CASCADE

The various proteins of the two complement pathways act in a sequence or cascade in numerical order except for C4. In the cascade, or series of steps, each protein activates the next one in the series, often by cleaving it. The resulting components have new functions. The classical pathway is initiated by the binding of antibodies to antigen, while the alternative pathway is initiated by cell-wall polysaccharides of the kind found in bacteria and fungi.

C3 has a major role in that it initiates several mechanisms that lead to microbial destruction. Both the classical and alternative pathways lead to the cleavage of C3 into fragments C3a and C3b. These initiate cytolysis, inflammation, and opsonization. The cascade of reactions culminating in these phenomena is illustrated in figure 5.1.

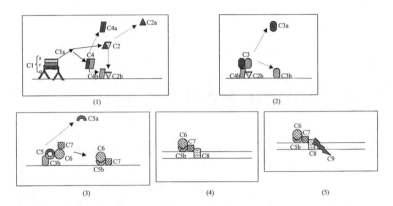

Figure 5.1. The classical pathway of complement activation leading toward cytolysis. (1) Activation of C1s by C1 interaction with the antibody. C1s then activates C4 and C2. C4a and C2a are released and C4b and C2b deposit on the cell surface, becoming the C3/C5 convertase. (2) C3/C5 convertase activates C3, releasing C3a and C3b deposition on the cell surface. (3) C4bC2bC3b then bind C5, cleave it, release C5a and deposition of C5b on the cell surface. C5b then binds to C6 and C7. (4) Binding of the C8 component, which is able to penetrate the plasma membrane and create small pores. (5) Binding and polymerization of the C9 component, completing the membrane attack complex and ultimately leading to lysis of the cell.

CYTOLYSIS

The most important function of the complement cascade is to destroy foreign cells. This is accomplished by damaging the cell membrane to the point that the cellular contents leak out. This process called cytolysis and the interactions involved are outlined in figure 5.1. The complement components C5 through C9 are referred to as the membrane attack complex (MAC), which produces transmembrane channels through the cell membrane leading to cell lysis or cytolysis.

INFLAMMATION

Components C3a and C5a contribute to acute inflammation. Their binding to mast cells, basophils, and blood platelets results in the release of histamine, which increases the permeability of blood vessels. C5a acts as a powerful chemotactic factor, attracting phagocytes to areas where complement has been fixed.

OPSONIZATION AND IMMUNE ADHERENCE

As shown in figure 5.1, component C3b coats foreign cells and can interact with special receptors on phagocytes to promote phagocytosis. This process is called opsonization. Additionally, C3b can coat particulate antigen that can then be bound by tissues that possess C3b receptors. This process is called immune adherence.

In order to prevent destruction of host cells, the destructive capacity of complement must be short-lived. Various regulatory proteins in the blood assure this short time of action by breaking down activated complement.

Various inherited deficiencies involving complement lead to diseases. For example, a deficiency of C3, which is rare, leads to greater susceptibility to bacterial infections; and deficiencies of C1, C2, or C4 cause collagen vascular disorders.

THE CLASSICAL PATHWAY

The steps involved in this pathway are shown graphically in figure 5.1.

Step 1: Activation of C1. The C1 component of complement is comprised of three parts C1q (hexamer), C1r (dimer), and C1s (dimer) held together by calcium ions. Activation of C1 is initiated by the binding of C1q to C1q-specific receptors on the Fc portions of adjacent (minimum two) antibodies. In humans, all antibodies have these receptors with the exceptions of IgG4, IgA, and IgE. Those antibodies possessing these receptors bind or "fix" complement. Those antibodies that do not possess these receptors and therefore are not able to bind complement, cannot fix complement. Once C1q has bound the C1q-specific receptors of two adjacent antibodies, it activates C1r, which in turn activates C1s. The activated C1s subcomponent then activates C4.

Step 2: Activation of C4. Although C4 is the second complement component of the cascade, it was the fourth complement component identified, and thus was denoted C4. The activated C1s activates C4 by cleaving it into two fragments, C4a and C4b. C4b binds to the surface of the cell membrane near the site of the antigen-antibody complex. Once bound to the surface, the C4b then binds the C2 complement component.

Step 3: Activation of C2. The C2 component is cleaved by the combined activities of C4b and C1s into C2a and C2b. The C2b portion remains attached to the C4b component on the cell membrane. Together the C4b-C2b complex is referred to as C3/C5 **convertase**. The C3/C5 convertase activates the C3 component of complement.

Step 4: Activation of C3. C3 is activated by the activity of C3/C5 convertase, which cleaves C3 into C3a and C3b. A single molecule of C3/C5 convertase is capable of activating hundreds of molecules of C3 and is thereby a means of amplifying the cascade by providing large amounts of C3a and particularly C3b. Both C3a and C3b have biological activity. C3a functions as an **anaphylatoxin**. C3b attaches to the cell membrane near the site of activation where it is capable of acting in immune adherence and/or opsonization. Some of the C3b combines with the C3/C5 convertase to form active C5 convertase, which activates complement component C5.

Formation of the membrane attack complex (MAC). This is formed as the result of the assembly and activation of complement components C5 through C9, and is the portion of the complement cascade that is involved in cytolysis of the target cell.

Step 5: Activation of C5, C6, and C7. C5 is cleaved by C5 convertase into C5a and C5b, both of which have biological activity. C5a functions as an anaphylatoxin and a **chemotaxin**. C5b binds C6 and C7 forming a complex that attaches to the surface of the target cell membrane.

Step 6: Activation of C8 and C9. The C8 component of complement then binds the C5b-C6-C7 complex on the cell membrane. This complex is capable of forming small pores in the membrane of the target cell, compromising its integrity. This is enhanced by the polymerization of the C9 complement component. The polymerization of C9 leads to the formation of transmembrane channels, culminating in target cell lysis.

THE ALTERNATIVE PATHWAY

The steps in this pathway are depicted graphically in figure 5.2.

The alternative pathway is initiated by the C3b component. The pathway is thought to be evolutionarily older than the classical pathway and does not require the formation of antigen-antibody complexes. Typically, this pathway is triggered by various substances including lipopolysaccharides (endotoxins) of gram-negative bacteria, **zymosan**, aggregated IgA, and a factor present in cobra venom. This pathway is

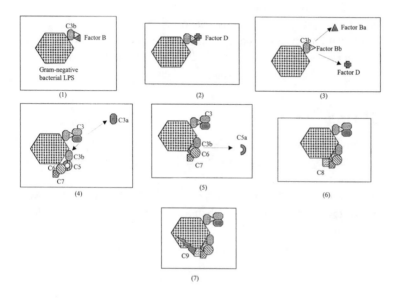

Figure 5.2. The alternative pathway of complement activation leading toward cytolysis. (1) Binding of C3b from the circulation to the surface of a bacteria cell. This in turn binds Factor B. (2) This complex is then bound by Factor D, which (3) cleaves Factor B, releasing itself and Factor Ba. Factor Bb remains bound to the C3b. (4) The Factor C3b/Bb complex then binds more C3 that it cleaves into C3a (released) and more C3b deposited on the bacterial cell surface. (5) C3b then binds C5, cleaves it, releases C5a and deposits C5b on the cell surface. C5b then binds C6 and C7. (6) Binding of the C8 component, which is able to penetrate the plasma membrane and create small pores. (7) Binding and polymerization of the C9 component, completing the membrane attack complex and ultimately leading to lysis of the bacterial cell.

possible due to the low levels of C3b present in normal serum, which can bind foreign antigens.

Step 1: Activation of factor B and factor D. Once C3b has bound a foreign antigen, it binds factor B in the serum, forming the C3bB complex. This complex is further activated by factor D, which cleaves factor B, resulting in the C3bBb complex. This complex functions as a C3 convertase, cleaving many molecules of C3. The C3b generated in the process is available to complex with more factor B in the serum, further activated by more factor D in the serum, thus amplifying the amount of C3 activation.

Step 2: The remainder of the pathway. At this point the classical and alternate pathways of complement activation are identical and proceed from C3b deposits on the cell surface, through the formation of the MAC, and ultimately the lysis of the target cell.

GLOSSARY

Anaphylatoxins—a group of substances that acts as mediators of inflammation. They are produced during the activation of the complement cascade.

Chemotaxin—a chemical stimulus responsible for the movement of cells.

Convertase—an enzyme that changes a substrate from one form to another.

Zymosan—an insoluble, mostly polysaccharide fraction of yeast cell walls.

CHAPTER 6

T Cell Receptors, Major Histocompatibility Complex, and Cytokines

Although these three molecules are discussed separately, their interactions are responsible for the immune response. Major histocompatibility complexes (MHC) are found on the surface of most body cells, indicating the cells belonging to "self." MHC molecules have the ability to bind small peptide fragments of antigens, and present those peptides on the surface of the cell for interaction with the appropriate immune cells.

The T cell receptors (TCR) are those molecules that recognize specific antigen in the form of short peptide segments bound to either MHC class I or class II molecules. If the TCR is able to bind antigen and the MHC molecule, this interaction leads to the production of specific cytokines that orchestrate the immune response to that particular antigen. It is this interaction that allows us to examine the TCR, MHC molecules, and the roles of various cytokines in the generation of an immune response.

T CELL RECEPTORS

The T cell receptor is a molecule on the T lymphocytes, which is able to specifically bind to antigen in association with the major histocompatibility complex. The TCR consists of **heterodimeric** glycopolypeptide chains linked together by **disulfide bonds**. These heterodimers allow the T-cells to recognize a heterogeneous array of protein antigens. As will be discussed in detail in chapters 7 and 8, the interactions of antigen presented by antigen presenting cells and the TCR are crucial to the formation and regulation of an immune response. Most human T cells express a TCR composed of an alpha/beta ($\alpha\beta$) heterodimer, while the remaining T cells have a gamma/delta (γδ) TCR. Both αβ and γδ TCRs are in noncovalent association with the polypeptides of CD3 (CD = cluster of differentiation). CD3 (also known as TCR signaling complex) is necessary for the expression of the TCR at the cell surface and is thought to be involved in **signal transduction** following antigen recognition by the TCR.

Structurally, the TCR resembles the Fab portion of immunoglobulins possessing N-terminal variable regions and C-terminal constant regions (see fig. 6.1). Both the variable and constant regions of the TCR are extracytoplasmic, followed by a transmembrane region and a short cytoplasmic region. Together, the TCR and the CD3 complex comprise what is referred to as the T cell receptor complex. The αβ TCRs are noncovalently linked to CD4 or CD8 molecules.

CD4 and CD8 are coreceptors or accessory molecules. These coreceptors divide αβ T cells into two major groups, CD4+ and CD8+ T cells. The coreceptors have two major functions. The first is they bind

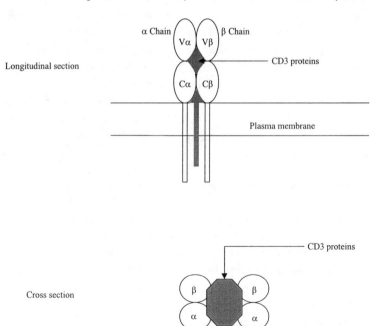

Figure 6.1. Longitudinal and cross sections of the αβT cell receptor

MHC molecules with low affinity. If the TCR recognizes the antigen in association with the MHC molecules, this binding is tightened, increasing the probability of stimulating an immune response. The αβ TCRs can ONLY recognize antigen in context of MHC molecules, not antigen alone. CD4 is capable of binding the invariant region of the MHC class II molecules, while CD8 binds the invariant regions of MHC class I molecules. The importance of these interactions will be described in chapters 7 and 8.

The second function of the coreceptors is that of signal transduction. The γδ TCRs, which are structurally similar to αβ TCRs, differentiate early in intrathymic development, and comprise a minority of TCRs. However, γδ TCRs can be found in great numbers in certain areas of the body. These include epithelial areas of the intestine, the uterus, and the tongue. In contrast with αβ TCRs, only some of the γδ TCRs are associated with the coreceptor CD8 and none have been identified in association with CD4. Therefore, the way in which γδ TCRs interact with antigen is different from that observed for αβ TCRs.

A great deal about the γδ TCR is not known, however there are several features that are known. The γδ TCRs are able to recognize N-formylated bacterial peptides, some mycobacterial antigens, self heat-shock proteins, or antigens in context of nonclassic MHC molecules such as CD1 in humans. However, once triggered, γδ T cells are able to release the same cytokines as αβ T cells and may also be involved in processes such as cytotoxicity. In general, it is thought that γδ T cells may have an early role in antimicrobial immune responses by recognizing self heat-shock proteins released by cells at infection sites and by responding to bacterial peptides themselves. In this manner, they are able to limit the infection until a specific αβ T cell response can be generated.

Gene Arrangement

The gene arrangement of the TCR α, β, and δ chains are shown in figure 6.2. The γ gene arrangement is very complex. The genes for the β and γ chains are found on different chromosomes, while the genes for the α and δ chains are found on chromosome 14 with the genes for δ being surrounded by those for α on both ends. Regardless, α and γ have V and J segments, which are rearranged in a manner similar to that of β gene locus

Vβ genes (1-range 50 to 100)	Jβ 1 genes (1-7)	Cβ1	Jβ 2 genes (1-8)	Cβ2

α and δ gene loci

Vα genes (1-100)	Vδ genes (1-3)	Dδ genes (1-2)	Jδ genes (1-3)	Cδ	Vδ4	Jα genes (1-100)	Cα

Figure 6.2. Genetic arrangement of the α, β, and δ TCR genes. The γ genetic arrangement is complex and therefore not included. Also not shown in this illustration are the noncoding regions between noted gene loci.

immunoglobulin light chains. The β and δ chains are composed of V, D, and J segments and are rearranged in a manner similar to the immunoglobulin heavy chains. In the germline, there are fifty to one hundred Vα and Vβ genes and five to ten Vγ and Vδ genes, which lead to part of the diversity necessary for interaction with many different antigens. The genetic expression of the TCR is also the same as that of the immunoglobulins, namely **allelic exclusion**.

Interestingly, the TCR gene rearrangement is a highly regulated event. In the germline cells, both rearrangements for the β and γ chains begin at nearly the same time. If the γ chain is successfully rearranged, then δ rearrangements begin. If the δ gene rearrangements are successful, able to be transcribed and translated into functional TCRs, a committed γδ TCR bearing T cell is formed. However, if the γ rearrangements are not successful, then the β rearrangements continue. The α rearrangements begin shortly thereafter. If these are successful, the result is an αβ TCR bearing T cell. If these too are unsuccessful, the result is apoptosis of the cell. The role of T cell receptors in the immune response is discussed in chapter 7, The Humoral Immune Response, and in chapter 8, The Cell-Mediated Immune Response.

MAJOR HISTOCOMPATIBILITY COMPLEX (MHC)

This is the collection of genes coding for the self-marking proteins or major histocompatibility complex, which was originally identified in investigation of transplantation rejection. These antigens occur on the surface of all the body's cells and identify them as belonging to the body and not foreign. Some MHC antigens appear on the surface of cells of the immune system. The human MHC region is known as the HLA (human leukocyte antigen) region and the corresponding genes are located on chromosome 6.

The MHC is subdivided into three regions known as class I, class II, and class III. Class I and class II are associated with the stimulation of T cells. Class III MHC contains an assemblage of twenty different genes, some cytokines, heat-shock proteins and complement factors. As only the MHC class I and class II antigens are associated with T cells, they will be the focus of this discussion.

MHC Class I Molecules

In humans, the class I genes contain three loci: A, B, and C. The analogous region in mice is K, D, and L. These genes encode a 43-kilodalton transmembrane protein that possesses three extracellular domains designated $\alpha 1$, $\alpha 2$, and $\alpha 3$ (fig. 6.3). These are in noncovalent linkage with a 12-kilodalton protein of $\beta 2$ microglobulin. The gene for this protein is located on another chromosome. The $\beta 2$ microglobulin is essential for the expression of the MHC class I molecule on the surface of the cell. In mice without a functional $\beta 2$ microglobulin gene, no MHC class I is expressed.

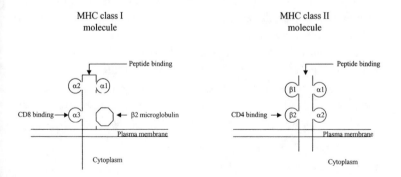

Figure 6.3. Diagrams of major histocompatibility (MHC) class I and class II molecules

MHC class I molecules are expressed on most of the nucleated cells of the body. This expression is such that all three class I molecules (A, B, and C) are expressed on the surface of cells simultaneously, known as coordinate expression. Additionally, MHC molecules are codominantly expressed, meaning that an individual expresses A, B, and C from the maternal parent and A, B, and C from the paternal parent simultaneously. Within an individual these molecules are always expressed and do not change. However, when we examine a population, we find that there are many stable alleles for MHC class I genes, a situation known as genetic polymorphism. For example, fifty HLA-B alleles have been identified and given the numbers HLA-B1 through HLA-B50. Comparing these alleles, one finds that they contain variable and invariable regions. When interacting with the TCR, the CD8 molecule interacts with the invariant region of the MHC class I molecule.

The cleft between the α1 and α2 domains of the MHC class I molecule is thought to be the peptide binding site for processed antigens (see chapter 7). The peptides interact with the variable regions of Vα and Vβ, which can accommodate a peptide approximately eight to nine amino acids in length. The interesting property of this site is that only peptides with specific key amino acids are able to bind this cleft. This is known as a binding motif; for example, HLA-A2 will only bind peptides that have a leucine in the second position and a valine in position 9. Processed peptides that do not have these key amino acids will not be presented to T cells by the HLA-A2. It is this binding that in part explains why not all antigens elicit a response from the immune system. Additionally, it partially explains why certain MHC profiles make an organism more susceptible or resistant to a particular disease.

Expression of the MHC class I molecule on the cell surface can be either upregulated (increased expression) or downregulated (decreased expression) by a variety of stimuli. For example, some viruses downregulate the expression of MHC class I molecules by infected cells, while the presence of interferon (IFN) γ upregulates expression of MHC class I molecules by cells.

MHC Class II Molecules

Like the MHC class I genes, the MHC class II region includes three genes. In humans these are DP, DQ, and DR. Each of these encodes an α chain and a β chain. Recent findings have indicated that there is more than one β chain associated with each of these genes and it is therefore possible that the same α chain can be associated with several different β chains. As the MHC class II molecules are also examples of genetic polymorphism and are codominantly expressed, this implies that an individual can express from ten to twenty MHC class II molecules on the appropriate cells. MHC class II molecules are expressed constituitively on B cells, dendritic cells, and thymic epithelial cells. The expression of MHC class II can be induced on other cells by IFN γ.

Structurally, the α and β chains of the MHC class II molecules are arranged as illustrated in figure 6.3. The peptide binding region is in the cleft formed between the α1 and β1 domains. With this arrangement, the MHC class II can interact with a peptide that is twelve to twenty-five amino acids in length, with the ends extending beyond the groove. Like MHC class I molecules, MHC class II molecules possess variant and invariant regions. The CD4 molecule of the TCR interacts with the invariant region of the MHC class II molecule.

Antigen Processing and Presentation

Antigen processing and presentation (see fig. 6.4) are crucial in determining which epitopes of a particular antigen will be targeted in an immune response. In general, exogenous antigens will become associated with MHC class II molecules, while endogenous antigens become complexed with MHC class I molecules. Although much of this area is still being investigated, the known basics are presented below.

Exogenous antigens will enter antigen-presenting cells (APCs) by phagocytosis. Peptide processing will begin when the phagosomes fuse with either endosomes or lysosomes. The enzymes associated with lysosomes then begin the breakdown of proteins into peptides and ultimately amino acids. At some point in the process, some of the peptides will be of the appropriate length (twelve to twenty-five amino acids) and binding motif to bind a MHC class II molecule. The MHC class II molecules are assembled and secreted via the secretory pathway (endoplasmic reticulum, to the **Golgi apparatus**, and released in vesicles) for expression on the cell surface. While still in the endoplasmic reticulum, the MHC class II molecules bind a self-peptide known as the

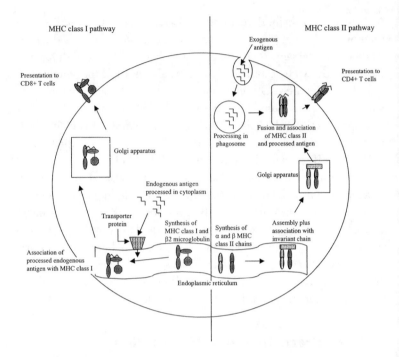

Figure 6.4. Antigen processing and presentation for both MHC class I (left) and class II (right) pathways

invariant chain. These MHC class II containing vesicles fuse with the phagolysome or phagoendosome. The invariant chains remain bound to the MHC class II molecules until exposed to the acidic pH of the phagolysosome, when they are released. The processed peptides of the correct size and binding motif bind the MHC class II molecules and are then transported to and expressed on the surface of the APC.

Endogenous antigens, such as viral antigens, are processed in either the endoplasmic reticulum or the cytoplasm. Those that are processed in the cytoplasm enter the endoplasmic reticulum via a transporter protein. Once in the endoplasmic reticulum, the processed endogenous antigens are available to interact with newly formed MHC class I molecules, which have already complexed with a molecule of $\beta2$ microglobulin. Those peptides of the appropriate length (eight to nine amino acids in length) and binding motif will bind with the MHC class I molecule and ultimately be transported to and expressed on the APC cell surface via the secretory pathway.

CYTOKINES

These are a diverse group of small (<30 kilodalton), soluble proteins produced by leukocytes that mediate a variety of immune functions. Those cytokines produced by lymphocytes are sometimes called lymphokines. Generally, they are secreted by one cell and bind to specific receptors on the corresponding target cell. Cytokines may also bind to the cells that produce them and have self-stimulation (autocrine) functions that result in such processes as cell division and protein synthesis and ultimately differentiation and clonal proliferation.

Those cytokines that mediate interactions between leukocytes are called interleukins (ILs). Most of the more than forty known cytokines are produced by either monocytes or helper T cells. The properties of some important cytokines are listed in table 6.1. Several cytokines in addition to the interleukins are included. They are IFN, interferon (see chapter 3); GM-CSF, granulocyte monocyte colony stimulating factor; and TNF, tumor necrosis factor.

In spite of the vast number of cytokines associated with the immune response, they have several features in common. They are antigen nonspecific glycoproteins that are rapidly secreted by the cells that produce them, rather than stored. Thus, they are very short-lived and are typically in minute quantities. These factors play a decisive role in the magnification of the immune response, from the interaction of a single cell with antigen to the precise interaction of many immune cells. These compounds are responsible for delayed-type hypersensitivity (DTH) responses (see chapter 10) and the recruitment of large numbers of monocytes to a site of infection. Each cell is capable of producing multiple cytokines and some of these overlap with regard to function, while each cytokine also has a unique function (see table 6.1). Each cytokine can affect many different types of cells, depending upon the cytokine receptors present on a particular cell.

Overexpression of cytokines can have a devastating effect on the immune response. Examples include the enterotoxin of *Staphylococcus aureus*, which can stimulate the Vβ of the TCR, which, in turn, leads to the massive release of cytokines associated with the **toxic shock syndrome**. Additionally, overproduction of TNFα by macrophages can lead to **septic shock**.

Table 6.1. Some Cytokines, Their Targets, and Immunological Effects

Cytokine	Synthesized by	Target	Primary effects
IL-1	Monocytes, macrophages, B cells, and others	T_H cells	Fever; activation of T_H2 cells
IL-2	T_H cells T_C and T_H cells	B cells	Proliferation of activated B cells T cell growth factor
IL-4	T_H cells and mast cells	Antigen primed/ Activated B cells	Activation/ proliferation/ class switching
IL-5	T_H2 cells	Activated B cells	Growth and Ig secretion
		Eosinophils	Growth and differentiation
IL-6	T_H cells and others	Proliferating B cells	Differentiation to plasma cells
IL-7	Fibroblasts, endothelial cells, and certain T cells	Pre-B cells Pre-T cells	Growth factor
IL-9	T cells	Mast cells	Activation
IL-10	T_H2 cells and macrophages	T cells macrophages	Inhibits T_H1 response; promotes T_H2 response
IL-12	B cells and macrophages	T cells NK cells	Inhibits T_H2 response; promotes T_H1 response; activates NK cells
IL-14	T cells	B cells	Differentiation to memory cells

(continued)

Table 6.1. (continued)

Cytokine	Synthesized by	Target	Primary effects
IFN-α	Leukocytes	Body cells	Antiviral activity
IFN-γ	T_H1 cells	Macrophages	Activation
		Body cells	Antiviral activity
		NK cells	Activation
		T cells	Inhibits T_H2 response
TNF-α	Monocytes, macrophages, and NK cells	Tumor cells and others	Cytotoxic, inflammation, fever, and septic shock
TNF-β	T cells	Tumor cells and others	Cytotoxic, inflammation
GM-CSF	Monocytes, macrophages, and T cells	Myeloid stem cells	Differentiation and growth of granulocytes and monocytes
M-CSF	Monocytes, macrophages, and T cells	Myeloid stem cells	Promotes monocyte/macrophage growth

GLOSSARY

Allelic exclusion—the situation observed with regard to gene rearrangement in germline T and B cells, where one chromosome is rearranged and prevents the use of the information on the second chromosome of the pair.

Disulfide bonds—these form as a protein folds to its native conformation. They stabilize the protein's three-dimensional structure.

Golgi apparatus—an assembly of vesicles and folded membranes in cells that receives, further modifies, and transports secretory products such as hormones and enzymes.

Heterodimer—a protein consisting of two polypeptide units; each of the subunits is different in its amino acid structure.

Septic shock—a disorder attributed to gram-negative bacteria and characterized by decreased blood flow, fever, rigors, impaired cerebral function, and, frequently, reduced cardiac output.

Signal transduction—the mechanism by which cells detect the presence of a ligand in the environment. This ligand binds specific receptors on the cell surface, which then stimulates signals for a specific response. Responses include cell division, secretion of specific proteins, and apoptosis.

Toxic shock syndrome—an acute and sometimes fatal disorder caused by streptococci and characterized by nausea, fever, diarrhea, and shock (reduced total blood volume and low blood pressure).

CHAPTER 7

The Humoral Immune Response

Humoral immunity, as stated earlier, is specific immunity mediated by antibodies. Antibodies or immunoglobulins are produced by plasma cells which are derived from B lymphocytes (B cells). Antibodies are found in the blood and tissue fluids of vertebrates and at particular times as much as 17 percent of the protein in blood consists of antibodies.

Figure 7.1 illustrates the relationship of humoral immunity and cell-mediated immunity. The latter is discussed in the next chapter.

STRUCTURE AND ASSEMBLY OF ANTIBODIES/IMMUNOGLOBULINS

The main structural features of the immunoglobulins are depicted in figure 7.2. Antibodies are glycoproteins made up of four polypeptide subunits connected by disulfide bonds. Two of these polypeptide subunits are referred to as heavy (H) chains with each having about four hundred amino acids. The other two, called light (L) chains, consist of about two hundred amino acids. The heavy chains are longer than the light chains and are similar with each immunoglobulin type (see below: Antibody/Immunoglobulin Type).

It was thought for many years that antibodies were derived from an inherited pool of genes. It is now known that the immune system has evolved a unique and ingenious method whereby each B cell assembles its own antibody genes *de novo* (afresh). Each B cell inherits several pools of gene fragments from which, as is shown in figure 7.2, it assembles a variety of antibody proteins.

The B cell inherits about three hundred small segments of DNA and from these it can assemble more than twenty thousand distinct antibody H-chain genes (see fig. 7.3). This is accomplished by the random but precise matching of their fragments. The number of different antibody proteins that can be produced is astronomical. This antibody variability far exceeds what is needed to cope with the myriad of antigens to which the vertebrate body is exposed.

The assembly of an antibody molecule is outlined below.

• As indicated in figure 7.2, antigen binds to the part of the antibody molecule at the end of each pair of H and L chains (Fab regions). The antigen-binding site varies between different antibody molecules but is identical for both halves of the same antibody molecule. The three dis-

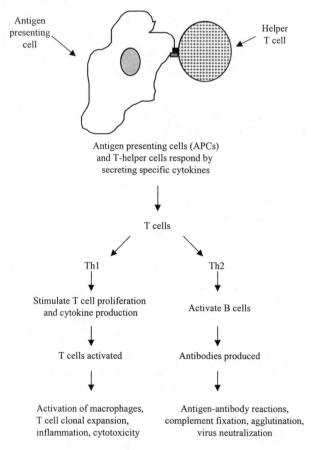

Figure 7.1. An overview of the specific immune response

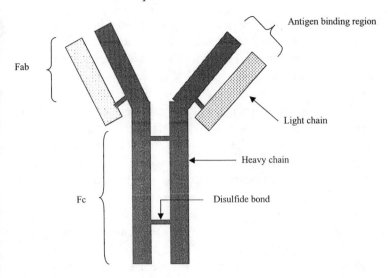

Figure 7.2. Generalized structure of the antibody

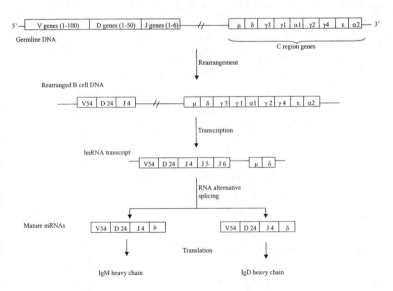

Figure 7.3. Gene arrangement of an antibody heavy chain

tinct parts, V, D, and J are involved in antigen-binding—parts V, D, and J with heavy chains, and V and J with light chains.

• As illustrated in figure 7.3, each of V, D, and J genes is encoded in the DNA as a distinct gene segment. With regard to the H chain, any V-gene segment can be combined with any D segment and this can be combined with any J segment, to produce the final antigen-combining region. In the same way an L-chain antigen-combining region is constructed by a random combination of a V- and a J-gene segment.

• The C regions are encoded by a separate set of genes and their role is to keep the antigen-binding sites properly oriented. The C region additionally can identify the L chains as both belonging to the kappa or lambda classes.

• With the H chains, the C region can identify the antibody as belonging to the IgM, IgG, IgA, IgD, or IgE isotypes. These regions do not vary appreciably between different molecules within a species.

ISOTYPE/CLASS SWITCHING

As illustrated in figure 7.4, mature B cells have on their surface IgM and IgD. However, secretion of the other antibody isotypes (IgA, IgG, and IgE) requires further rearrangement of the DNA. In the absence of antigen, little to no class switching takes place. In the presence of specific antigen a series of events leads to the final rearrangements of the antibody molecule. It is to be emphasized that the portion of the antibody molecule that has been rearranged to interact directly with the antigen has occurred in germline cells. Class switching is a phenomenon associated exclusively with the 5' end of the constant portion of the heavy chain genes (see fig. 7.3).

A mature B cell encounters antigen that is bound by the antigen-binding portion of the surface IgM or IgD antibodies. The bound antigen is internalized by the B cell and partially degraded. Some of the degraded antigen is associated with MHC class II molecules and is ultimately presented to CD4+ T cells. This interaction leads to activation of the T cell, which then begins secreting cytokines in response to the interaction with the antigen. This, in turn, activates the B cell to undergo alternative splicing and secrete a particular isotype of antibody with the exact same antigen specificity as occurred on its surface. Once com-

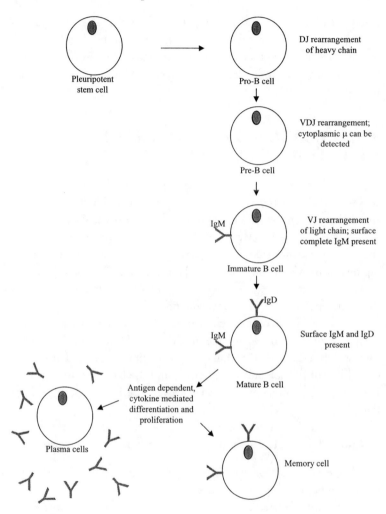

Figure 7.4. B cell maturation and differentiation

pleted, the B cell has successfully transformed to a plasma cell, secreting specific antibody.

The isotype of antibody that will be ultimately secreted is dependent upon the cytokines present as the result of interaction with the T cell. In mice, when IFNγ is present, the antibody secreted is of the IgG2 isotype. In both mice and humans, the presence of IL-4 stimulates a class switch to IgG4 or IgE. There is much more to be elucidated as to which cytokines direct specific isotype switches. The isotype of antibody present also influences the success or failure of a particular immune response.

THE CLONAL SELECTION THEORY OF ANTIBODY PRODUCTION

The most important evolutionary development of the immune system of vertebrates was the capability of generating millions of different specificities of antibody. This is done blindly (mechanism explained below) without any knowledge of the antigens, microbial or otherwise, that may be encountered. This capability was necessary because of the rapidity with which microbes can change genetically. As will be discussed later, vertebrates have evolved a system for mutating their genes that is independent of sexual reproduction.

Since the time of Ehrlich (early 1900s) various theories have been put forward to explain the production of antibodies. A theory now widely accepted, the clonal selection theory, evolved from the early ideas of Ehrlich and Landsteiner, and the later contributions of Pauling, Jerne, Talmadge, and Burnet over a period of about twenty-five years.

The final form of the clonal selection theory of antibody production is attributed to MacFarlane Burnet. The theory posits the following:

• A special subset of cells in each animal is responsible for antibody production.

• The antibody-producing cells, the B lymphocytes, are the basic units of this system. They produce one and only one antibody. Each cell has the capacity to produce a different antibody, and it displays a copy of that antibody on its surface.

• This antibody is generated randomly without reference to the vast antigenic universe. When a given cell is stimulated via its surface antibody, production of that antibody follows.

• In addition to stimulating the start of antibody production, the cell is stimulated to divide and produce large numbers of clonal progeny all of which can produce the same antibody. The progeny cells live on after the initial antibody production.

• Any clones produced that cross-react with self molecules are eliminated (anergy) so as to avoid an autoimmune response.

The hypothesis just outlined accounts for the three principal features of the immune system: diversity, **tolerance** of self, and memory.

Diversity

This is the number of different B cell receptors or the different antibodies the variable region sequences produce in a particular animal species. It is also called the repertoire and each vertebrate creature has the ability to generate a complete antibody repertoire, which is present at birth.

Tolerance of Self

It was proposed that clones of antibody-producing cells reactive to self would have to be eliminated; however, many antiself clones are not eliminated but are kept under control. The term "negative selection" refers to the deletion of self-reactive B lymphocytes and self-reactive T lymphocytes as they develop in the thymus. Alternatively, some cells are in a state of unresponsiveness called **anergy**. Although still present, they are unable to respond to antigen by a variety of mechanisms; in contrast, deletion results in **apoptosis** and elimination of the cell.

Memory

Much about the development of memory cells is unknown. However, several aspects of the generation of memory B cells have been elucidated. The purpose of developing memory B cells is to generate a faster and more intense immune response to a particular antigen upon second exposure. This phenomenon has been exploited in vaccine development; the better the vaccine, the more memory cells produced in response to that antigen or antigens.

Memory B cells have several characteristics that can be used to differentiate them from other B cells. These cells are nonproliferating and are very long-lived. They reside primarily in the germinal centers of secondary lymphoid tissues. In contrast with immature and mature B cells that express IgM and/or IgD on their surface, memory cells are IgG+/IgA+. They also express a high concentration of **CD44** on the surface, which allows for localization in the secondary lymphoid tissues. The precise stage where memory cells develop is not known. However, plasma cells do not become memory cells.

The basics of the process start with the activation of mature B cells by specific antigen. These cells are stimulated to differentiate and proliferate in response to various cytokines. During this process, some of the cells become memory cells for that particular antigen.

ANTIBODY RESPONSE AND ANTIGEN-ANTIBODY INTERACTIONS

Most antigens (small molecules and soluble proteins) are thymus dependent; that is, they require help from T cells to initiate antibody formation by B cells. In order to elicit antibodies, a thymus-dependent antigen must be taken up and processed by an antigen presenting cell (APC).

The processing involves enzymatic degradation of the antigen and its linkage to a MHC class II molecule that has been synthesized in the APC (see chapter 6). The combination of the processed antigen and the class II molecule is presented at the surface of the APC to a helper T cell.

The helper T cell recognizes and binds to the combination, the processed antigen binding to the T cell receptor (TCR). This initiates production of the cytokine **interleukin**-1 (IL-1) by the APC. IL-1 has many effects, including lymphocyte activation. The helper T cell, in response to this interaction, secretes IL-4, IL-5, and IL-6. These cytokines are responsible for cell division and differentiation of the reactive B cells, having antigen on their surface. Some of these B cells become plasma cells, which first secrete specific antibodies of the IgM class and later specific antibodies of the IgG class (see fig. 7.4).

Some reactive B cells become memory cells that produce little or no antibody. These cells are able to react to any subsequent exposure to the original antigen. The antibody response to a subsequent exposure is more vigorous and is referred to as the anamnestic response.

In some instances, memory cells are not formed to thymus-dependent antigens. An example is the lack of memory cells formed in response to the capsular polysaccharide of *Haemophilus influenzae* type B. This failure is due to the immaturity of the B cells in newborns and infants, who may sustain serious infections by the aforementioned bacterium.

Some antigens do not need T cell help in order to stimulate antibody production by B cells. These are the T-independent antigens. These antigens are typically of bacterial origin, high molecular weight with repeating antigenic determinants, and are resistant to degradation. Examples are lipopolysaccharide and bacterial flagellin.

PRIMARY AND SECONDARY HUMORAL IMMUNE RESPONSES

Primary Response

The primary response refers to the response generated by a first encounter with a particular antigen. This primary response is subdivided into four phases: latent phase, exponential production phase, steady state, and the declining phase (see fig. 7.5).

In the latent phase, there is the initial encounter with an antigen. Seven to fourteen days later, antibody (typically IgM) can be detected. The time lapse in this phase is related to the time necessary for antigen processing, presentation to T cells, proliferation of specific B cell clones, and secretion of detectable antibody levels in the bloodstream. The exponential production phase is characterized by the exponential increase in the amount of antibody present in the bloodstream. Steady state is achieved when the production and degradation of the circulating antibody are essentially equal. The declining phase is the result of the shut down of the immune response and a rapid decline in the amount of circulating antibody, typically within a few weeks.

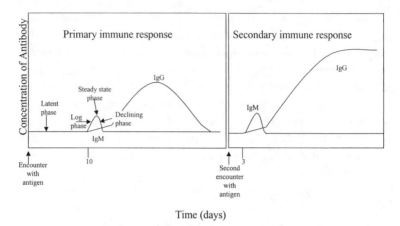

Figure 7.5. Dynamics of the primary and secondary immune response upon an initial and a second exposure to a particular antigen

Secondary Response

The secondary response refers to the response generated by a second exposure to the same antigen. In this case, the memory cells generated in the primary response help mediate the secondary immune response, which is much quicker and of greater magnitude (see fig. 7.5). To this end, the latent phase is of lesser time, the amount of antibody secreted is greatly increased, and the production of antibody may continue for longer periods of time—months or even years.

In contrast with the primary immune response, the secondary response is characterized by a shift in the class of antibody being made from IgM to IgG. The IgG is in much greater quantity than IgM and appears for a longer time. In addition, IgA and IgE antibodies may also be present. The switch to IgG has several effects on the immune response. IgG is capable of activities including neutralization of **endotoxins**, activation of complement (except IgG4), and opsonization. It is the most stable of the antibody **isotypes** in the bloodstream with a half-life of twenty-three days. Last, IgG is able to cross the placental barrier and passively transfer maternal immunity to the unborn mammal.

GLOSSARY

Anergy—the phenomenon whereby lymphocytes that have been primed by an antigen fail to respond on second contact with the antigen.

Apoptosis—a form of programmed cell death characterized by the fragmentation of nuclear DNA.

CD44—a type 1 transmembrane protein that is found in many tissues and on many cell types.

Endotoxin—a complex lipopolysaccharide (LPS) molecule composing the cell wall of some bacteria.

Immunological tolerance—a state of nonreactivity to antigen that ordinarily would induce humoral or cell-mediated immunity. Immune tolerance may be produced in adults from administration of large or small amounts of antigen or contact with antigen in fetal or early postnatal life.

Interleukin—small molecular weight glycoproteins secreted by leukocytes that affect other leukocytes, and thus modulate an immune response.

Isotype—when applied to immunoglobulins it describes the immunoglobulin class, immunoglobulin subclass, light chain type and subtype. It can also apply to the variable region.

CHAPTER 8

The Cell-Mediated Immune Response

Unlike humoral immunity, cell-mediated immunity (CMI) cannot be transferred from the immunized animal to a naive animal with anti-serum (antibodies). However, it was learned that CMI could be transferred from animal to animal when certain lymphocytes were transferred. This cellular immunity is specific (natural killer cells excepted) and mediated by T lymphocytes that recognize MHC-bound antigens. The important features of the relationship between CMI and humoral immunity are shown in figure 7.1.

Immunity to those diseases caused by obligate intracellular pathogens (e.g., viruses), facultative intracellular parasites (e.g., *Mycobacterium tuberculosis*), some bacteria, fungi, protozoans, and helminths is primarily cell-mediated. Generally speaking, immunity to a particular bacterial pathogen is predominantly humoral or cell-mediated, although both are involved.

T LYMPHOCYTES (T CELLS)

T cells are the main component of CMI and, like B cells, they are derived from precursor stem cells in the bone marrow. As stated in chapter 2, the precursor lymphoid stem cells develop into natural killer cells and T cells. The T cells further differentiate in the thymus.

There are four main types of T cells, all of which produce various cytokines (discussed in chapter 6) after stimulation by antigen. The cell origin, target cells and effects of cytokines are summarized in Table 6.1.

The T cells discussed below have surface antigens that make possible their identification.

The natural killer cells and four kinds of T cells are as follows:

Natural killer (NK) cells. These lymphocytes, which were discussed in
   chapter 2, are neither T cells nor B cells, but are of lymphoid line-
   age. They are able to kill tumor and virus-infected cells without specific antigen stimulation. Like cytotoxic T cells they use perforin to
   lyse target cells. The cells they attack frequently have reduced or
   altered MHC class I expression.

Cytotoxic T (Tc) cells. Tc cells are involved in killing foreign cells. These
   cytotoxic T cells recognize foreign antigens imbedded in MHC class
   I molecules. They possess the surface antigen CD8 and produce the
   cytokine gamma interferon. After contact, Tc cells are able—with
   the protein perforin (a pore-forming protein)—to destroy cells of
   neoplasms and transplant tissue by apoptosis (nonnecrotic cell
   death). They are also able to lyse and kill some virus-infected cells.
   Tc cells are only effective in killing cells containing foreign antigen.

Helper T (Th) cells. These cells have a surface antigen called CD4. Th
   cells are required for the production of normal levels of antibody by
   B cells and they aid in the development of CMI. The various functions of Th cells are due to cytokines interleukin (IL)-2 , IL-4, IL-6,
   IL-10, and gamma interferon. See table 6.1 for the target cells and
   their effects. Two subsets of Th cells referred to as Th1 and Th2,
   which have different functions, are discussed below.

Delayed hypersensitivity T (Td) cell. These lymphocytes have the surface
   antigen CD4 and are considered to be a subset of the Th cells mentioned above. CMI can be transferred with these lymphocytes. They
   produce several cytokines whose functions include attracting
   macrophages and other defensive cells. Td cells are also involved in
   the rejection of transplant tissue, some allergic reaction, and immunity to neoplasms.

Suppressor T (Ts) cells. Refers to T cells that serve to produce cytokines
   and other effects that suppress the immune response. Markers to
   identify a true Ts subset have yet to be identified.

The CMI response can come about in two basic ways, by the T-
independent mechanism or the T-dependent mechanism. The T-independent mechanism is of primary importance in the immune response
during the time it takes the body to generate a T-dependent response.

In the T-independent mechanism, microbial structures that are present early in an infection are recognized. These structures include the formyl peptides of bacteria and bacterial LPS. These substances have direct effects upon the immune system. Many of these compounds are chemotactic, recruiting various immune cells to the site of infection, particularly phagocytes. For example, endotoxin can activate the alternative complement pathway and thus potentiate the release of chemotaxins C3a and C5a. Additionally, these compounds can stimulate the release of cytokines from macrophages and other cells. For example, endotoxin can bind to specific receptors on leukocytes, stimulating the leukocyte to secrete cytokines that recruit more leukocytes to the site of infection.

In the T-dependent mechanism, the role of T cells is decisive in determining the overall immune response toward a particular antigen. The "decision" of T cells is largely influenced by the profile and quantities of cytokines present at the site. Of central importance is the Th subset of T cells, which will modulate the various cell responses associated with an "appropriate" immune response. This, in turn, will generate various profiles of cytokines in the area leading to delayed-type hypersensitivity (DTH) and various immunopathologic effects, even immune suppression.

As illustrated in figure 8.1, the interaction between the Th cell and the antigen presenting cell (APC) orchestrates the remainder of the immune response. The APC will determine which epitopes are targets of the immune response, based upon those that are capable of being presented with the MHC class II molecule. The response of the Th cell will translate into one of three possible effector mechanisms: cytotoxicity, macrophage activation by Th1 cells, or antibody production by Th2 cells. Dedication of the immune response to the "wrong" mechanism will ultimately lead to enhanced susceptibility to that particular antigen. The ability to stimulate the "right" immune response is often the test of the efficacy of a newly developed vaccine.

CELL-MEDIATED CYTOTOXICITY

Discussion of the CMI deals with the various mechanisms associated with cell-mediated killing of target cells, such as tumor cells or virus-

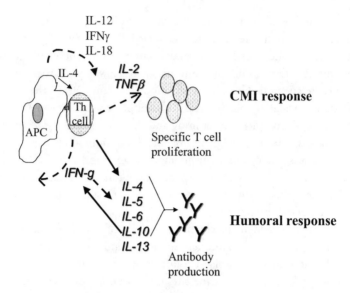

Figure 8.1. The central role of the helper T cells in the development of the immune response. Th1 responses are indicated by dashed lines, Th2 by solid lines. Decision toward Th1 or Th2 responses is based upon the interaction of the Th cell with the APC, in this case a macrophage. In a Th1 response, this interaction stimulates the production of IL-2 and gamma interferon by the Th cell. Gamma interferon activates the macrophages, enhancing their ability to destroy foreign cells. IL-2 promotes the proliferation of specific T cell clones in response to the invader. IL-12 secretion aids in promotion of the Th1 response. Gamma interferon suppresses the IL-10 and thereby "turns off" the Th2 response. If the interaction of the Th cell and the APC results in the Th2 response, the cytokines released by the Th cell are those that promote maturation of specific B cell clones to become plasma cells and secrete antibody. The presense of IL-10 suppresses secretion of gamma interferon and thus "turns off" the Th1 response.

infected cells. The primary cells associated with cell-mediated cytotoxicity are Tc cells and NK cells. Tc cells recognize target cells, typically those that are virus-infected, by antigen bound to the MHC class I molecule. NK cells recognize those cells that fail to express MHC class I molecules on their surface as potential targets. Some viruses, such as herpesviruses, downregulate expression of the MHC class I molecule on the surface of the host cell. Although the cell is no longer a target for Tc cells, it is now a target for NK cell killing.

The killing mechanisms by Tc cells and NK cells are similar and fall into one of three basic mechanisms: direct cell-cell interactions, cytokine-mediated, and granule-mediated. Direct cell-cell interactions involve interaction with Fas (CD95). The Fas ligand (Fas L) is expressed on the surface of mature, activated CD4+ and CD8+ T cells. Fas interaction with FasL stimulates intracellular signaling events that lead to apoptosis of the infected cell. Cytokine-mediated killing is very similar to cell-cell killing, except that it is based upon cytokines, such as TNF, binding their receptor on target cells, the TNF receptor. These interactions also lead to signaling mechanisms that result in death of the target cell.

Cell killing based upon the release of granules is very different from the other two mechanisms. It involves interaction between the target cell and either the Tc or NK cell in order to stimulate the release of granules by the Tc or NK cell. The granules are contained in vesicles that fuse with the plasma membrane of the Tc or NK cell and release their contents into the space between the Tc or NK cell and the target cell. The granules contain several proteins, including perforins and granzymes. Perforin is a pore-forming protein that requires the presence of calcium in order to polymerize and form transmembrane channels in the plasma membrane of the target cell. Perforin alone can cause lysis and death of the target cell by compromising the integrity of the target cell plasma membrane. The Tc and NK cells are unaffected by perforin as they possess a proteoglycan, chondrotin sulfate A, which inactivates the perforin. Granzymes are a collection of serine proteases. They pass into the target cell via the transmembrane channels created by the perforin where they interact with the various intracellular pathways that trigger apoptosis and DNA degradation. Granzymes are not required for cytotoxicity.

Another method of cell-mediated cytotoxicity, which is essentially a variation of the granule mechanism described above, is known as antibody-dependent cell-mediated cytotoxicity (ADCC). This mechanism is commonly used against large pathogens, such as helminths. A specific immune response is mounted against the target, which becomes coated with specific antibodies. The Tc or NK cells are triggered to release their granules by binding the Fc portion of the antibodies. The remainder of the mechanism is the same.

THE ROLE OF MACROPHAGES

Macrophages have a role in all phases of the immune response. As illustrated in figure 8.2, macrophages are involved in the initial defense of the host by engulfing microbes and in response to the latter, secreting cytokines that attract more phagocytes to the area. Macrophages function as APCs that determine the epitopes available to T cells that ultimately decide the immune response toward a particular antigen. Macrophages are effector cells in CMI, and once activated by cytokines present in the area, they serve to produce additional cytokines, in addition to antitumor and antimicrobial activities. Last, macrophages play crucial roles in inflammation, fever, tissue reorganization, and tissue repair.

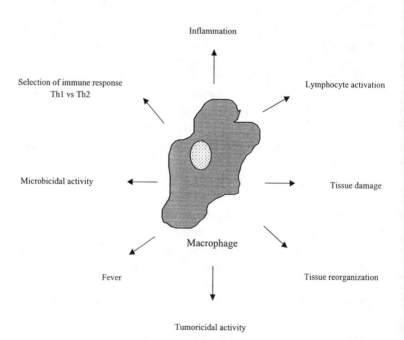

Figure 8.2. The central role of macrophages in many aspects of the immune response

IMMUNOPATHOLOGY

The immunopathology associated with the CMI falls into four basic categories:

• The first is chronic inflammation. The immune response is directed against self-antigens or **commensal** organisms resulting in inflammation that damages the surrounding tissue. This is observed in rheumatoid arthritis, **Crohn's disease**, **sarcoidosis**, psoriasis, and multiple sclerosis.

• The second category is cytotoxicity. The immune system destroys virus-infected cells, sometimes killing cells that are necessary for the survival of the host, such as brain cells.

• The third category is excessive cytokine release, which causes the immunopathologic changes associated with toxic shock syndrome and hemorrhagic necrosis.

• The last category is granuloma formation. Failure of the CMI response to eliminate bacterial or fungal parasites and foreign or other antigenic material (lacking solubility), often results in the formation of granulomas. T cells continue to be recruited to the site of the offending antigen and continue to release cytokines that recruit more leukocytes to the area. The granuloma begins with proliferation and aggregation of macrophages, eventually consisting of an accumulation of epitheloid cells, multinucleate giant cells along with activated macrophages and sometimes a necrotic center. It ultimately consists of a nodular mass of varying size. Granulomas vary in character depending upon the antigen involved. Some of the diseases in which granulomas occur are tuberculosis, syphilis, histoplasmosis, blastomycosis, leprosy, and schistosomiasis. Although they are defensive in nature by sequestering the infection, they may through their size and location, contribute to symptoms. Granulomas may also occur in some autoimmune diseases.

GLOSSARY

Commensalism—a parasitic state in which the organism lives in or upon its host without causing disease. The organism benefits from the relationship but the host may or may not.

Crohn's disease—a disease mainly affecting the small intestine (regional ileitis) and characterized by cramps, diarrhea, local abscesses, weight loss, and inappetance. The cause is not known.

Sarcoidosis—a disease of unknown cause characterized by nodules mainly in the lymph nodes, skin, lungs, and bones.

CHAPTER 9

The Immune System in Action

IMMUNITY TO BACTERIA

Bacteria are a diverse group of small, unicellular, ubiquitous organisms. They are prokaryotes (no distinct nucleus) that occur widely in nature and in association with animals and humans. Contrary to popular belief, only a relatively small number are capable of causing disease.

Specific and nonspecific mechanisms are involved in the body's defense against pathogenic bacteria. The six nonspecific mechanisms are discussed in chapter 3. In summary, they are:

• The skin and other epithelial surfaces are not penetrable by most bacteria, and fatty acids on the surface of the skin are toxic to many bacteria. The skin also has antiviral properties, including enzymes that break down RNA viruses.

• The ciliary action of the trachea, coupled with mucus, removes bacteria, and the flushing of urine removes many bacteria from the urinary tract.

• Phagocytosis (nonimmune), the engulfment and destruction of bacteria, and other foreign material by macrophages and neutrophils, is a major defense mechanism.

• **Commensals** of the normal flora occupy niches on the skin and other epithelial surfaces that prevent pathogenic bacteria from becoming established. An example is lactobacilli on the mucous membrane of the vagina.

• The acidity of the stomach and vagina prevents the establishment of potentially harmful bacteria.

• Defensins are a family of small peptides that constitute about 30 percent of granule-associated proteins of neutrophils; they are also found in macrophages. They kill bacteria and fungi by binding to their membranes and increasing membrane permeability.

The fate of bacteria that penetrate the barriers of the skin and other epithelial surfaces depends largely on the immune response. The following eight features of bacteria contribute to their survival and capacity to produce disease:

- There are differences in the cell wall of the four following broad categories of bacteria, **gram-positive**, **gram-negative**, mycobacteria (cause tuberculosis, leprosy, etc.), and spirochetal organisms (cause leptospirosis, syphilis, etc.).
- Cell wall: Gram-positive bacteria have a cell wall outside their plasma membrane that is composed of peptidoglycan. The host's enzyme lysozyme (in tears, saliva, etc.) acts on the links of N-acetyl muramic acid-N-acetyl glucosamine in the peptidoglycan layers. The outer layer of the cell wall of gram-negative bacteria consists of lipopolysaccharide (LPS, also called endotoxin), a complex lipid structure. This is affected by pH, the high salt concentration of sweat, and the presence of short chain fatty acids.
- Capsules: Most are composed of large polysaccharide molecules; some, such as the plague and anthrax bacteria, have protein capsules. Capsules are antiphagocytic and thus contribute to virulence; they are also poor activators of the alternative complement pathway.
- Flagella: These are responsible for motility and possess antigenic proteins that in the case of some gram-negative enteric (intestinal) bacteria (e.g., *Salmonella* spp.) are highly antigenic.
- Pili: These very small filamentous structures resemble flagella but are not involved in motility. They enable bacteria to adhere to host cells.
- Toxins: Exotoxins are those released extracellularly. Most are produced by gram-positive bacteria and some, such as botulinus and tetanus toxin (associated with botulism and tetanus, respectively), are highly toxic. In general, exotoxins are destructive to phagocytes, local tissue, and, in some instances, the central nervous system. The exotoxins produced by some gram-negative bacteria, for example, some strains of *Escherichia coli*, are less toxic. Endotoxin or LPS is released when gram-negative bacteria disintegrate. It can be toxic and deleterious to the host in a number of ways. Enterotoxins refer to those toxins that act on the tissues of the gut. Some enterotoxins are known to stimulate the overproduction of cytokines resulting in shock syndromes.

• Some species of mycobacteria (the cause of tuberculosis, leprosy, etc.) have very strong cell walls that are rich in lipids. This enables them to resist intracellular killing and thus survive in macrophages as intracellular parasites.

• The spirochete of syphilis attempts to mimic host antigens and by this stratagem escapes actions of the immune system. Other spirochetes also have the ability to vary surface antigens to confuse the antibody-forming system, such as in relapsing fever (*Borrelia hermsii*, in the United States).

In brief, the antibacterial role of antibody is as follows:

• Antibody to pili, some capsules, and lipotechoic acid block attachment of the bacterium to the host membrane.

• When bacteria proliferate they initiate complement-mediated injury to gram-negative outer lipid layers.

• Specific antibody directly blocks bacterial surface antigens that interfere with microbial nutrition.

• Antibody to M proteins (some streptococci) and capsules opsonize the bacteria via Fc and C3b receptors for phagocytosis.

• Bacterial **immunorepellents**, which are toxic for leukocytes and interfere with normal phagocytosis, are neutralized by antibody.

• Bacterial toxins and spreading factors (e.g., **hyaluronidase** of streptococci), which contribute to the invasion of and spread within tissues, are neutralized by antibody.

Eventually most bacteria are killed by phagocytosis. The processes are briefly as follows:

• Chemotaxis: Various bacterial and complement components (e.g., C5a) attract phagocytes.

• Attachment of bacteria to the phagocytic surface via a receptor on the macrophage membrane.

• For various reasons, not all bacteria are taken up by phagocytes and not all organisms taken up trigger killing mechanisms.

• When inside the phagocytic cell, lysosomes fuse with phagosomes to form phagolysosomes and killing mechanisms are initiated. Details of the phagocytic process are described in chapter 3.

• Phagocytes have a number of complex oxygen and nonoxygen dependent mechanisms for killing bacteria. They vary with the kind of phagocyte and also with different bacteria.

• Mycoplasmas are spherical to filamentous bacteria that lack a cell wall. They cause a number of subclinical or chronic infections. *Mycoplasma pneumoniae* causes a widespread disease of humans called primary atypical pneumonia. These organisms elicit IgM antibodies followed by IgG and secretory IgA, which are important in the host's resistance. The significance of cell-mediated immunity in mycoplasmal infections is not clear.

• Chlamydiae are small, obligately intracellular, gram-negative bacteria that cause mainly subclinical to chronic infections. *Chlamydia psittaci* causes the important **zoonotic** disease psittacosis. Antibodies are produced in response to (result of) chlamydial infections, but they do not prevent reinfection of the individual. The precise role of cell-mediated immunity has not yet been determined.

• Rickettsiae are small, obligate intracellular, gram-negative bacteria that comprise several genera and a number of species. They cause the well known typhus fevers and Rocky Mountain spotted fever of humans. Cell-mediated immunity is more important in resistance than humoral immunity.

IMMUNITY TO VIRUSES

Viruses are very small infectious agents that invade and reproduce in eukaryotic and prokaryotic cells. They have no cell wall and no independent metabolic activity. Their genome may be either DNA or RNA (either single or double stranded) and it is surrounded by a protein coat. The DNA genomes may be linear or circular helices. Viruses cannot reproduce outside the host cell. Instead, they co-opt the host cell's reproductive machinery for transcription, translation, and replication. New viruses are released from the host cell, which may be destroyed in the process. Some viruses spread directly from cell to cell rather than by a **viremia**. The resultant infections may be acute (lytic) or the virus remains dormant and persistent (lysogenic). In the case of lysogenic viruses, subclinical infections are sometimes reactivated to cause clinical disease. Some of the important human viral diseases and their causal viruses are listed in table 9.1.

Table 9.1. Some Important DNA and RNA Viruses Causing Disease in Humans

Viral family	Examples	Diseases
DNA viruses		
Adenoviridae	Serotypes 1–48 and others	Upper respiratory tract infections, in general
Hepadnaviridae	Hepatitis B virus	Hepatitis B, hepatocellular carcinoma
Herpesviridae	Herpes simplex 1 and 2, varicella-zoster, cytomegalovirus, Epstein-Barr, human herpes viruses 6, 7, and 8	Herpes simplex, chickenpox, shingles, cytomegalic inclusion disease, Burkitt's lymphoma, nasopharyngeal carcinoma, oral and genital herpes
Papovaviridae	Papilloma virus	Warts, skin, and cervical cancers
Poxviridae	Variola, vaccinia	Smallpox, cowpox
RNA viruses		
Arenaviridae	Lymphocytic choriomeningitis viruses, Lassa virus	Lymphocytic choriomeningitis, Lassa fever and other hemorrhagic fevers
Bunyaviridae	Hantaviruses	Hantavirus cardiopulmonary syndrome, hemorrhagic fever with renal syndrome
Filoviridae	Ebola virus, Marburg virus	Ebola hemorrhagic fever, Marburg hemorrhagic fever

(continued)

Table 9.1. (continued)

Viral family	Examples	Diseases
RNA viruses		
Flaviviridae	Genus *Flavivirus* viruses	Yellow fever, Dengue fever, hepatitis C
Orthomyxoviridae	Influenza viruses	Influenza
Paramyxoviridae	Genus *Morbillivirus* viruses	Mumps, measles
Picornaviridae	Enterovirus, rhinovirus, hepatovirus	Gastroenteritis, polio, coxsackie, hepatitis A, "common cold"
Reoviridae	Rotavirus	Respiratory and gastrointestinal infections, Colorado tick fever
Retroviridae	Human T-lymphotrophic virus, human immuno-deficiency virus	Adult leukemia, tumors, AIDS
Rhabdoviridae	Lyssavirus	Rabies
Togaviridae	Rubella	Rubella (German measles)

Immunity to viruses involves the following:

• Interferon comprises a group of proteins produced by the cell in response to viral infection that protects the cell from infection (see fig. 9.1).

• Viral antigens are largely protein or glycoprotein. The immune response to viral antigens is mainly T cell dependent, including the antibody response.

• Specific antibody prevents entry and viremic spread of some viruses; it also recognizes virus-infected cells. IgM and IgG are important in plasma and tissue fluids; IgA protects epithelial surfaces.

• It is of interest that the antibody-forming system in responding to the altered self antigens may produce antiself antibodies (autoantibodies) that can be important in autoimmune disease.

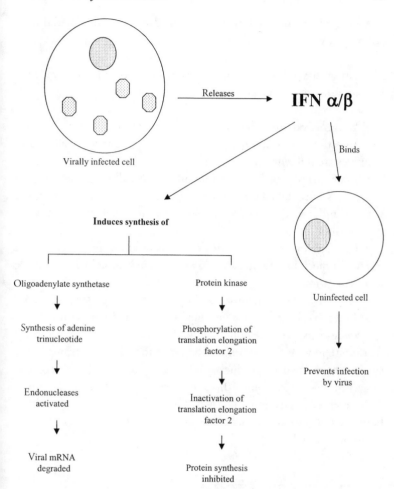

Figure 9.1. The molecular action of interferon in viral infection

• Antibody and complement (C1-C9) can directly affect enveloped viruses and cause lysis of virus-infected cells.
• Cytotoxic T cells can recognize altered self MHC class I antigens and respond to these, in addition to viral antigens, on the cell surface.
• Natural killer cells are effective in killing those virus-infected cells with lesser or no MHC class I on the surface.

• The role of delayed type hypersensitivity in viral infection is still controversial.

Viruses have a variety of mechanisms that allow them to evade the host immune response. These include:

• Antigenic variation that is the result of mutation, allowing for multiple infections with different variants of the same virus. Well-known examples are influenza and cold viruses.
• Some viruses, such as the human cytomegalovirus, possess glycoproteins with IgG-Fc receptor binding activity, which interferes with complement activation and blocks the attachment of antiviral antibodies.
• The Epstein-Barr virus and adenovirus produce short segments of RNA that block interferon activation of protein **kinases**, which impede viral replication.
• Some viruses encode proteins that inhibit the expression of MHC class I on the cell surface, e.g., adenovirus and cytomegalovirus.
• Some viruses encode homologs of cytokines and cytokine receptors that interfere with the immune response to the virus; for example, the shope fibroma virus produces a homolog of the TNF receptor. However, when TNF binds this homolog, the function of the TNF-TNF receptor interaction is blocked. The Epstein-Barr virus produces a homolog of IL-10; however, the immunological consequence of this has yet to be clarified.

IMMUNITY TO FUNGI

Fungi are eukaryotic cells (distinct nucleus) that exist as single cells or a multicellular mycelium that is composed of filamentous structures or hyphae. They do not possess chlorophyll and their cell walls consist primarily of chitin. Some have capsules and, although some are associated with humans, the majority are saprophytes found in the soil and on decaying vegetation.

The immune response to fungi is poorly understood. In general, the immune processes that protect humans from bacterial infection are similar to those that protect humans from fungal infections. In general, an effective immune response against fungi is cell-mediated. As with bacteria, there is considerable variation in responses with different fungi. Fungal infections can be classified as follows:

Superficial: Dermatophytosis (ringworm) is caused by filamentous fungi that live off skin, hair, and nails by feeding on their keratin. *Candida albicans*, a yeastlike commensal fungus, causes infections of the skin and mucous membrane (particularly of the mouth and vagina) called candidiasis.

Subcutaneous: These infections are initiated by trauma, and the fungi involved are saprophytes. The infections are characterized by the formation of chronic nodules and ulcers.

Systemic or respiratory: These diseases are usually subclinical lung infections due to saprophytic fungi such as *Histoplasma capsulatum* (histoplasmosis) and *Blastomyces dermatiditis* (blastomycosis). These infections for various reasons, including impaired immunity, can become disseminated and life threatening.

Some of the important aspects of immunity to fungal infections are as follows:

• Normal individuals are able to resist serious fungal infections; however, those whose cell-mediated immunity is impaired are much more vulnerable.

• Infections with dermatophytes are relatively mild and self-limiting in normal individuals. Resistance is based largely on the cell-mediated response; affected individuals develop a delayed-type hypersensitivity response to fungal antigens.

• It has been shown that some yeasts activate complement by the alternate pathway.

• T cell immunity is involved in resistance to most fungal infections and T cells release lymphokines that activate monocytes and macrophages to destroy fungi.

• In those diseases in which granuloma develop, protective immunity depends upon cell-mediated immunity. Humoral immunity has little if any protective role. The number of granulomas and their size reflects the individual's immune status.

IMMUNITY TO PROTOZOA AND HELMINTHS

The protozoa and the helminths are much larger than bacteria and viruses, which translates into an increased variety and quantity of antigens available for interaction with the immune system of the host. As a result, there are many features of the immune response to these organisms that are common to both groups. For example, many effector cells aid in the elimination and control of parasites. They include macrophages, neutrophils, eosinophils, and platelets. All of these are capable of releasing reactive oxygen intermediates and nitric oxide in order to eliminate the parasite. The responses by these effector cells are enhanced by the presence of specific cytokines. T cells are central to the immune response against parasites. However, antibodies are effective against extracellular parasites, particularly IgE and IgG.

These parasites also share commonality in mechanisms for evasion of the host immune response. These include:

• Antigenic variation.
• Complex life cycles with stage-specific antigen profiles.
• The release of "free antigen" allowing the organism to become established while the immune system is "busy" responding to extraneous antigens.
• The formation of protective cysts.
• Antigen masking in which the parasite covers itself with host antigens.

Protozoa

Protozoa are eukaryotic (have a distinct nucleus) microorganisms that comprise a diverse group of single-celled, animal-like organisms that are considerably more complex than prokaryotes, such as bacteria. About twenty protozoans are pathogenic for humans. They cause such diverse diseases as amoebic dysentery, malaria, and sleeping sickness.

Important features that enable protozoans to survive are the following:

• Some are spread by insects.
• Some have an intracellular habitat and thus can conceal antigens.

• Some are capable of antigenic variation and immunosuppression. In what is called antigen masking, some parasites cover themselves with host antigens.

Most parasites are well adapted and as a result, acquired immunity against them is seldom complete. What immunity there is, called **premunition**, is effective in keeping most infections subclinical.

Protozoa elicit both humoral and cell-mediated responses. Humoral immunity is active against parasites that are free in the circulation and tissue fluids, while cell-mediated immunity is directed mainly against intracellular protozoans. Antiparasite antibodies may agglutinate and opsonize protozoa, and along with complement or cytotoxic T cells, may aid in killing them.

Pathogenic protozoans have a considerable capacity to resist the immune system. *Giardia lamblia*, an intestinal protozoan, can cause chronic diarrhea in humans; the carrier rate (no evidence of clinical disease) for this widespread organism may be as high as 20 percent. Secretory IgA and IgM antibodies against *G. lamblia* are found in the small intestine of infected individuals; however, these antibodies directed to flagella and attachment disks of *Giardia* are thwarted by the frequent change in the parasite's surface antigens.

African sleeping sickness is caused by *Trypanosoma gambiense* and *T. rhodesiense*, both of which are transmitted by tsetse flies. These protozoan flagellates are also able to change their surface antigens. The coat of these protozoans consists of a single protein called variable surface glycoprotein (VSG), which can be altered by a single gene. These trypanosomes have genes for as many as a one thousand variants of VSG.

Immunosuppressed individuals become susceptible to protozoans that ordinarily reside in the host in a subclinical, quiescent state. *Pneumocystis carinii*, which lives quiescently in human lungs, can become pathogenic when the immune system is suppressed by the human immunodeficiency virus (HIV). The cyst forms of the ordinarily subclinical protozoans *Cryptosporidium* and *Toxoplasma* can give rise to disease if immunity is impaired.

Interestingly, the resistance of humans to the trypanosomes of rodents is attributed to high-density lipoprotein (HDL), which agglutinates them. This is a clear example of natural immunity.

In view of the ways that protozoans can circumvent host defenses and survive, the possibilities for the development of effective vaccines are not particularly sanguine. However, there has been some progress made toward a malarial vaccine for humans, and vaccines have been developed for the prevention of diseases due to protozoan blood parasites in domestic animals.

In some cases, host resistance to certain protozoans appears to be genetic. Certain HLA antigens endogenous to West Africans have some correlation with protection against severe malaria. Additionally, other populations in Africa do not possess the Duffy antigen on the surface of their erythrocytes. As this antigen is the means by which *Plasmodium vivax* gains entry to the erythrocytes in its life cycle, those individuals not possessing the Duffy antigen are naturally immune to malaria caused by this parasite.

Helminths

Helminths include nematodes (roundworms), cestodes (tapeworms), and trematodes (flatworms). Some important helminths and associated diseases are as follows:

NEMATODES (ROUNDWORMS)

There are numerous diseases associated with nematodes. Some of the better known are:

• *Ascaris lumbricoides*: This large, intestinal roundworm infects mainly children and occurs worldwide.
• Guinea worms: Adults live under the skin and can reach four feet in length.
• Hookworms: May cause severe anemia.
• *Trichinella spiralis*: The cause of trichinosis in humans, a disease most frequently acquired by consuming parasitic cysts in insufficiently cooked pork.
• Filarial worms: These very small nematodes (microfilariae) cause elephantiasis and "river blindness" in some tropical regions.

TREMATODES

These flat worms spend part of their life cycle in snails from which cercariae (larvae) infect humans. The principal disease they cause is schistosomiasis, which occurs widely in the tropics.

CESTODES

The adults of a number of species of tapeworms live, usually harmlessly, in the intestine of humans and animals. Disease is caused when tapeworm larvae develop and produce cysts in various tissues including the brain and liver (echinococcosis).

The kinds and forms of helminth parasites are remarkably varied and thus the immune responses are very complex and incompletely understood. The feature that appears to be the most important in the elimination or control of helminths is the production of IgE. This is coupled with the activity of eosinophils that are stimulated to degranulate in an ADCC manner and kill the parasite by cytolysis.

IMMUNITY TO TUMORS

Cancer is the uncontrolled growth of body cells. Growth inhibitory factors control the growth of most cells. A number of characteristics distinguish cancer cells from normal cells. For instance, cancer cells are nutritionally less fastidious than normal cells and require fewer growth factors. This allows them to grow profusely resulting in masses of varying size, called tumors. Benign tumors are ones that the body can wall off and thus are noninvasive. In contrast, malignant tumors are invasive and destructive of normal tissues and organs. Some malignant tumors, in a process called metastasis, spread to other parts of the body and initiate new tumors. The term "neoplasm" (new growth) is used to denote both benign and malignant tumors.

The growth and division of normal cells is controlled by at least two kinds of genes. Protooncogenes promote growth, but are controlled by growth-restraining tumor-suppressing genes. Changes in both of these kinds of genes can result in unregulated cell growth that may lead to cancer. Carcinogens (certain chemicals), ultraviolet and ionizing radiation,

X-rays, and certain viruses may alter some of the these genes resulting in cells becoming cancerous. At one stage a protooncogene may become an oncogene (a gene whose expression causes formation of a tumor). Some cancers that may be caused by viruses are listed in table 9.2.

Neoplasms are very heterogeneous and different kinds of tumors elicit different immune responses. In general, antigens associated with tumor cells are weak.

Tumor Antigens

Some features of tumor antigens are:

• Tumor cells may lose their histocompatibility and blood group antigens.
• Cells of colon carcinomas may lose their capacity to produce mucus.
• Tumor cells may acquire new antigens.

Table 9.2. Viruses Associated with Human and Animal Cancers

Cancer	Virus
Human:	
Adult T-cell leukemia	Human T-cell leukemia virus, Type D (Retrovirus)
Burkitt's lymphoma (B cell)	Epstein-Barr virus (Herpes)
Cervical cancer	Papillomavirus (Papovavirus)
Hepatocellular carcinoma (Liver cancer)	Hepatitis B virus (Hepadnavirus)
Nasopharyngeal carcinoma	Epstein-Barr virus (Herpes)
Animal:	
Bovine leukosis	Bovine leukosis virus (Retrovirus)
Feline leukemia	Feline leukemia virus (Retrovirus)
Marek's disease of chickens	Herpesvirus

• Embryonic antigens that are absent from normal cells may be reexpressed when cells become malignant.

• Some human neoplasms have antigenic proteins ordinarily found only in the fetus.

• The carcino-embryonic antigen (CEA) associated with tumors of the intestinal tract is normally found in the fetus. The fetal antigen alpha-fetoprotein is produced by hepatoma (cancer of the liver) cells.

• The stem-cell antigen of acute lymphoblastic leukemia is characteristic of one stage in the maturation of lymphocytes. This antigen is rare in differentiated lymphocytes.

• Tumors induced by viruses tend to acquire antigens characteristic of the virus.

• Tumors induced by chemicals have cells that carry new surface antigens.

Immune Responses

Tumor cells differ antigenically from normal cells and thus are considered foreign and are attacked. The principal mechanisms involved are those of natural killer NK cells and cytotoxic T cells. Macrophages are involved usually to a lesser extent.

Natural Killer Cells

These cytotoxic lymphocytes are found in relatively small numbers in the blood, secondary lymphoid organs, and bone marrow. They recognize and rapidly kill (cytolysis), nonspecifically, a variety of sensitive tumor cells, **xenogeneic cells**, and some virus-infected cells.

Natural killer (NK) cells are regulated by cytokines and have receptors for interleukin-2 and interferons (IFN). All three interferons (alpha, beta, and gamma) increase NK cell function.

NK cells that show an enhanced capacity to kill both tumor cells and virus-infected cells have been referred to as LAK (lymphokinase activated killer) cells. They are activated by cytokines such as interleukin-2.

Macrophages

Activated macrophages kill tumor cells directly. They are also thought to be part of a surveillance system against the development of tumors.

Tumor destruction is contact-mediated and nonphagocytic. Macrophage secretions involved in destruction are lysosomal enzymes, proteases, hydrogen peroxide, and tumor necrosis factor.

T Cell-Mediated Immunity

A cell-mediated response to tumor antigens can occasionally be demonstrated by *in vitro* tests and skin tests (delayed-type hypersensitivity). Cytotoxic T cells can frequently be demonstrated *in vitro* from individuals with tumors. However, it is thought that T cell–mediated immunity is mainly important in the control of tumors induced by viruses. ADCC (antibody-dependent cell-mediated cytotoxicity) is also important in the regression of tumors.

Humoral Immunity

Antibodies to tumor antigens are found in many individuals with tumors. In conjunction with complement they are thought to be mainly effective against free cells, such as metastasizing cells and leukemic cells. It would appear that antibodies have little effect on solid tumors.

Immunosuppression

It is well known that individuals with neoplasia are often severely immunosuppressed. Generally speaking, tumors involving T cells suppress cell-mediated immunity, while B cell tumors suppress the humoral or antibody response. This immunosuppression is observed to be as much as one hundredfold greater in the B and T cell malignancies. Increased incidence of immunosuppression is observed in radiation victims and in individuals who are intentionally being immunosuppressed, as well as older individuals with decreased immune responsiveness. The actual mechanism is currently unclear.

In addition to immunosuppression, other mechanisms by which tumors evade the immune system include:

• Tumor localizing in an immunologically sequestered site where it is not in contact with immune cells.

• Antigenic modulation whereby the tumor cells either change or lose surface antigens.

• Release of tumor-specific or associated antigens. These "free antigens" now work as described for protozoans and helminths.

• Nonspecific suppression initiated by **prostaglandin** synthesis by the tumor cells.

• Large tumor masses provide an overwhelming amount of antigen for the immune system, thus rendering the immune response ineffective.

TUMOR IMMUNOTHERAPY

Various immunological means have been, and are being used, to treat cancer. Some of these are discussed below.

Nonspecific Immune Stimulation

The attenuated vaccine strain of *Mycobacterium bovis* (**BCG**) is the most widely used immune stimulant. BCG has a nonspecific, positive effect on cell-mediated immunity by activating macrophages and natural killer (NK) cells. It is given systemically by injection or inoculated directly into the neoplastic mass.

Other nonspecific immune stimulants include a bacterial vaccine prepared from *Proprionobacterium acnes* (used like BCG), **levamisole**, and thymus hormones. Vaccines consisting of gram-negative bacteria contain endotoxin, which stimulates the production of tumor necrosis factor by macrophages. This factor interferes with the blood supply to tumors and activates macrophages and NK cells.

The interferons have been effective against **hairy cell leukemia**, but have had little influence on other tumors. Interleukin-2 and LAK cells have led to the regression of melanoma and renal carcinoma.

Tumor Infiltrating Lymphocytes

Tumor infiltrating lymphocytes (TIL) are lymphocytes that are removed from a biopsied tumor. Like LAK cells, these are exposed to IL-2 *in vitro* and injected into the tumor. TILs appear to have a greater specificity for tumor cells than LAK cells and may therefore be a more promising candidate for tumor immunotherapy.

Adoptive Immunotherapy

This involves the passive transfer of immunity from one individual to another with lymphocytes. In animals it has been shown that the adoptive transfer of tumor "immune" lymphocytes mediates antitumor effects on neoplasms. In humans this would involve the culture, *in vitro*, of large numbers of specific T cells using IL-2.

Passive Immunotherapy

This involves the use of monoclonal, antitumor antibodies, to cause tumor regression. Among the disadvantages of this approach is the fact that tumor epitopes occur on other cells. Also, to be at all effective the tumor must be well vascularized.

Another approach that has shown some promise is the use of immunotoxins, a combination of a **monoclonal antibody** and a toxic agent. The antibody is targeted to the cancer cell and the attached toxic agent destroys it without damaging healthy tissue. Among the toxic agents that have been conjugated to monoclonal antibody are ricin (from the castor bean), chlorambucil (from nitrogen mustard), and radioisotopes.

Bone marrow transplantation to irradiated **leukemic** patients is an example of immunodepletive therapy. After irradiation with or without chemotherapy to destroy leukemic cells, patients are given a bone marrow transplant (stem cells) from healthy donors. Such transplants may generate serious graft versus host reactions. An alternative approach is to remove some **autologous** bone marrow from the patient before irradiation and/or chemotherapy. This bone marrow material must be purged of tumor cells before being returned to the patient. Autologous bone marrow transplants have been effective against several cancers including **lymphoma** and T cell leukemia.

Cytokine Immunotherapy

This refers to the use of a variety of cytokines (IFN α, β, and δ, IL-1, IL-2, IL-4, IL-5, IL-12, and TNF), which either singly or in combination, stimulate tumor regression. To date this type of immunotherapy is inconclusive.

GLOSSARY

Autologous—this denotes derived from self.

BCG—Bacille (Bacillus) Calmette-Guérin (French researchers).

Commensalism—a parasitic state in which the organism lives in or upon its host without causing disease. The organism benefits from the relationship but the host may or may not.

Gram-positive, gram-negative—the Gram stain is widely used in the identification of bacteria. With this procedure some bacteria remain violet colored (gram-positive) and some are decolorized (gram-negative). Gram-positive and gram-negative bacteria differ in the structure and composition of the cell wall.

Hairy cell leukemia—a leukemia characterized by an enlarged spleen and an abundance of large mononuclear cells whose irregular surface projections give a flagellated or hairy appearance.

Hyaluronidase—this enzyme breaks down and thus lowers the viscosity of hyaluronic acid, a mucopolysaccharide that is an important constituent of tissues.

Immunorepellents—bacterial immunotoxins that are specifically toxic for leukocytes.

Kinase—an enzyme that catalyzes the transfer of phosphate groups from ADP or ATP to a substrate.

Leukemia—an acute or chronic neoplasm characterized by an abnormal increase in the number of leukocytes. It is classified according to the kind of leukocyte most prominently involved.

Levamisole—a drug used as an anthelmintic (mainly against nematodes) and also in cancer therapy.

Lymphoma—a malignant tumor of lymphoid tissue.

Monoclonal antibody—a single type of antibody, produced by a hybridoma cell line, and directed against an antigenic determinant (epitope). The hybridoma cell line is formed by the fusion of a lymphocyte cell and a myeloma cell (from a plasma cell cancer).

Premunition—a state of protective immunity that occurs when small numbers of pathogenic microorganisms, especially blood-borne protozoans, persist within the host.

Prostaglandins—a number of hormonelike compounds that have a variety of functions as inflammatory mediators.

Viremia—the presence of virus in the host's blood.

Xenogeneic cells—grafted tissue derived from species different from the recipient.

Zoonotic—diseases that are capable of being transmitted from animals to humans.

CHAPTER 10

Hypersensitivity Reactions, Part I: Allergy and Anaphylaxis

Although the immune system is generally protective and beneficial, it can on occasion malfunction and give rise to immune disorders. Some of these disorders, known as hypersensitivity reactions, are the result of an exaggerated immune response, mediated by either antibodies or immune cells. The four different types of hypersensitivity reactions are types I, II, III, and IV. This chapter will focus on type I hypersensitivity reactions. Hypersensitivity reaction types II, III, and IV will be discussed in chapter 11.

TYPE I IMMEDIATE OR ANAPHYLACTIC HYPERSENSITIVITY

In this hypersensitivity reaction antigen combines with IgE antibody fixed on mainly mast cells and basophils resulting in the release of vasoactive substances, such as histamine. This type of hypersensitivity is characterized by rapid (within minutes) onset of symptoms following reexposure to antigen. Allergic reactions to ordinarily innocuous antigens, such as pollen, are typical examples of type I hypersensitivity. Anaphylaxis is an acute form of allergy.

ALLERGY AND ANAPHYLAXIS

Allergy and anaphylaxis result from type I immediate hypersensitivity. Anaphylaxis is a rare, life-threatening, acute form of allergy. The term "anaphylaxis" was introduced by Paul Portier and Charles Richet (1902) in explaining results of their investigation into the mechanism of marine invertebrate poisons on mammalian physiology. In their experiments, dogs were injected with Mediterranean sea anemone toxin.

Several weeks later a minute amount of the toxin was injected as a "booster shot" for the dogs. However, instead of increased resistance against the toxin, the dogs showed a variety of symptoms including increased salivation, diarrhea, difficulty breathing, paralysis of the hind limbs, and death within minutes. To describe this phenomenon, Portier and Richet used the term "anaphylaxis," from the Greek *ana* meaning away from and *phylaxis* meaning toward protection. This was the first example of the immune system being harmful rather than beneficial for the individual.

Generally in allergy, certain antibodies, or reagins, react with certain allergens or antigens to produce a number of deleterious reactions that result in such diseases as asthma, eczema, hay fever, and urticaria (hives). In rare instances the reactions may lead to anaphylaxis. It is estimated that one in five individuals suffer from allergies.

Allergens have many sources including plants; fungi; pollen and fungal spores; house mites; foods such as milk, eggs, and cereals; insect venom; drugs; and animal dander. Ordinarily innocuous substances that should be ignored by the immune system are instead deemed a potential hazard and therefore stimulate an immune response.

The German investigators Prausnitz and Kustner demonstrated in 1921 that the agent that caused immediate hypersensitivity circulated in the blood. The skin test they used developed into a technique for the routine screening for allergy to specific substances in humans. This test for skin sensitivity, which is still used, is referred to as the P-K test. It had been shown earlier that hypersensitivity could be transferred to an unsensitized animal with serum from the hypersensitive animal (passive transfer).

Development of Allergy

Steps involved in the development of allergy are as follows and as shown in figure 10.1:

• The allergen may be inhaled, ingested, or taken in through the skin via injuries or insect bites. Repeated application to the skin of certain chemicals may cause allergic contact dermatitis or allergic eczema (see below).

• After the allergens enter the vascular system they are engulfed by phagocytes, which carry them to B lymphocytes.

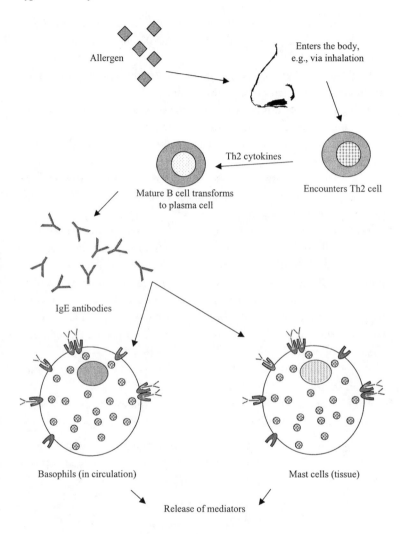

Figure 10.1. Basic features of the allergic process. An allergen enters the body and subsequently encounters a Th2 cell. This interaction stimulates the liberation of Th2 cytokines, which activates the appropriate B cells to produce IgE to the antigen. The IgE enters circulation and binds to the IgE Fc receptors on the surface of basophils and mast cells. Subsequent encounters with antigen will stimulate degranulation and the release of mediators, such as histamine, leukotrienes, and prostaglandins.

• The B cells are activated in response and differentiate into plasma cells that secrete specific antibodies (reagins) called immunoglobulin E (IgE).

• IgE in blood circulates throughout the body. The IgE level is low in the normal animal, but can be elevated in the allergic state.

• The body does not react harmfully on initial exposure to the allergen; hypersensitivity occurs on subsequent exposures.

• It is not known why individuals are allergic to a particular antigen and not others.

• Type I immediate hypersensitivity results from the reaction between allergen and IgE on the surface of basophils and mast cells. IgE may be present on these cells indefinitely.

• The attachment of IgE (Fc portion) to the cell membranes sensitizes the basophils and mast cells. This sensitization may last for weeks and even years and thus subsequent exposure to the particular allergen may initiate an allergic reaction. Reactions may range from mild to severe.

• When the allergen contacts the sensitized cell a chemical signal triggers the release of granules from these cells. These granules accumulate in various tissues and release inflammatory mediators, including chemotactic factors, into blood.

• The result is an acute inflammation initiated by an allergen rather than an injury.

• IgE is selectively produced in helminth (parasitic) infections and individuals with helminth infections have higher levels of IgE.

There are three phases associated with the allergic response: the sensitization phase, the activation phase, and the effector phase. Occasionally there is also a late phase reaction.

THE SENSITIZATION PHASE

Approximately 50 percent of the population produces IgE antibodies to airborne allergens, such as pollen. Of those, only about 10 percent have clinical symptoms. The reason for this is multifactorial. The production of IgE antibodies by B cells is T cell dependent, specifically upon the production of IL-4 by CD4+ Th2 cells. It takes repeated exposure to the airborne allergen to produce sufficient quantities of specific IgE to develop clinical symptoms. This threshold effect is what is most likely the rationale behind the statement that people develop allergies with age. With time there are potentially more encounters with the offending allergen. The development of the IgE response defines a person as sensitized.

The IgE antibodies are then released into circulation where they rapidly attach to basophils and mast cells via IgE-specific Fc receptors. These Fc receptors have a very high affinity for IgE. Therefore, once the IgE has bound to the receptor it persists on the cell surface for several weeks. The cell remains sensitized as long as the antibody remains bound on the surface.

THE ACTIVATION PHASE

This phase is initiated by reexposure to the offending allergen (sometimes referred to as a challenge dose). In an anaphylactic reaction, the peak response will occur within ten to fifteen minutes and then wane. What has actually transpired is that at least two IgE Fc receptors have been cross-linked (see fig. 10.2). This cross-linking results in receptor aggregation, stimulating the methylation of membrane phospholipids resulting in a change in membrane fluidity. This change in fluidity allows for an influx of calcium ions, which stimulates **exocytosis** of the granules and the production of prostaglandins, thromboxanes, and leukotrienes. The extent to which a particular basophil or mast cell degranulates is not an "all or nothing" phenomenon; a cell can exocytose some or all of its granules, depending upon the amount of receptor cross-linking, reform granules, and repeat the process. Concomitant with the influx of calcium ions is a drop in intracellular **cAMP** levels, which also favors calcium entry into the cell and degranulation.

THE EFFECTOR PHASE

This is the phase associated with the pharmacological activity of the substances released by degranulation as well as those produced *de novo* (afresh).

Among the preformed mediators are:

Histamine. This is the principal mediator. It binds to two different receptors called H1 and H2. The H1 receptors are located on

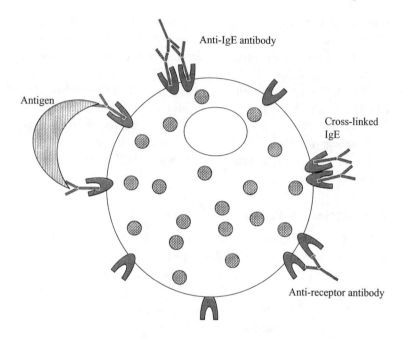

Figure 10.2. Ways that IgE receptors on basophils and mast cells can be cross-linked

endothelial cells (cells lining blood vessels). It causes capillaries to enlarge and become permeable resulting in loss of fluid and production of a characteristic rash. If the loss of fluid is great, shock may result from the drop in blood pressure. Histamine also binds to the H1 receptors associated with smooth muscle of the upper respiratory tract, bronchi and bronchioles. These are stimulated to contract leading to breathing difficulty and asthma. Histamine binds to H2 receptors associated with the smooth muscle of the gastrointestinal tract, stimulating release of stomach acid from the stomach mucosa resulting in cramps and severe diarrhea. Last, histamine binds the H2 receptors that stimulate nasal mucous secretion or increased vascular permeability, depending upon the location of the H2 receptor. H1 receptors can be blocked by antihistamines; however, these have no effect on the H2 receptors. The blocking of H2 receptors requires H2 receptor antagonists such as cimetidine (trade name Tagamet).

Chemotactic factors. The neutrophil chemotactic factor and eosinophil chemotactic factor-A attract neutrophils and eosinophils, respectively.

Serotonins. These are responsible for smooth muscle contraction and increased vascular permeability in some species, such as rodents.

Bradykinin. A vasoactive **nonapeptide**, whose action is similar to that of histamine but slower; it is present in the blood during anaphylaxis.

Platelet activating factor. This activates platelets to release mediators (histamine and serotonin, in some species), which may result in microthrombus formation. Platelet activating factor is the most potent cause of bronchoconstriction and vasodilation known. It is capable of inducing shock symptoms within minutes in extremely low doses.

Heparin. Heparin is an acidic proteoglycan (mucopolysaccharide) that makes up the matrix holding the basic mediators such as histamine and serotonin within the granules. With degranulation and release of mediators, heparin inhibits coagulation. This mediator is not directly involved in anaphylaxis.

Among the *de novo* mediators are:

Leukotrienes. Derived from mast cells with actions similar to histamine. Some have chemotactic factors for neutrophils and eosinophils. These de novo mediators are present in extremely small quantities and promote prolonged smooth muscle constriction.

Prostaglandins and thromboxanes. Derived from mast cells with action similar to histamine. These mediators are vasoactive and promote bronchoconstriction, as well as being chemotactic for a variety of white blood cells, including neutrophils, eosinophils, basophils, and monocytes.

Cytokines. These proteins, described in detail in chapter 6, are made and secreted by various cells and act as intercellular mediators that have a variety of effects on cells.

THE LATE PHASE REACTION

This reaction is the result of inflammatory responses mediated by the accumulation of neutrophils, eosinophils, basophils, lymphocytes, and macrophages. The congregation of a large percentage of activated eosinophils and neutrophils intensifies the type I hypersensitivity reactions. The late phase reaction follows the anaphylactic reaction within four to eight hours and can persist for several days.

One portion of the late phase reaction involves the interaction of thromboxanes, IL-3, IL-5, and eosinophil chemotactic factor-A. These mediators stimulate further eosinophil degranulation, result-

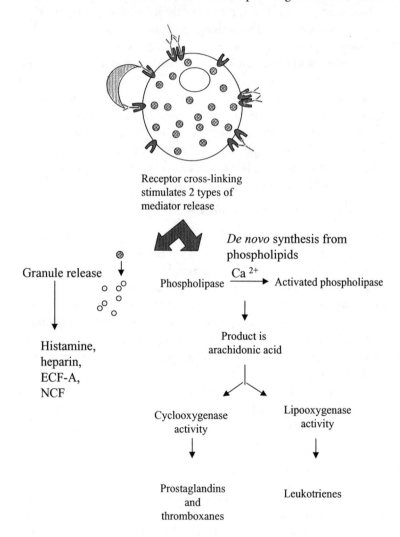

Figure 10.3. Origins of mediators released as a result of IgE receptor cross-linking

ing in the release of leukotrienes, platelet activating factor, histamine, arylsulfatase, major basic protein, and eosinophilic cationic protein. The combined actions of leukotrienes, platelet activating factor, histamine, and arylsulfatase result in local tissue damage. Major basic protein leads to the destruction of various parasites, such as schistosomes (trematodes), by affecting their mobility and inflicting surface damage. However, major basic protein is also extremely toxic to the mammalian respiratory tract, resulting in tissue damage. Eosinophilic cationic protein is an antihelminth mediator, containing a neurotoxin and an helminthotoxin, which also inflicts tissue damage in the host.

The actions of neutrophil chemotactic factor and IL-8 combine to stimulate activation, phagocytosis, and degranulation of neutrophils in the late phase reaction. These lead to the release of lysosomal enzymes, leukotrienes, and platelet activating factor, all of which cause tissue damage. Additionally, the combined actions of these mediators are chemotactic for T cells, B cells, and macrophages. These responses are protective when the host is confronted with a parasitic infection, but damaging when stimulated by an innocuous substance such as pollen.

Allergic Contact Dermatitis/Allergic Eczema

A wide range of compounds including formaldehyde, plant resins (poison ivy, poison oak), aniline dyes, cosmetics, insecticides, and heavy metals have been implicated in allergic contact dermatitis. This form of allergy may occur after repeated application of these chemicals. These compounds act as haptens when they bind covalently or noncovalently to self proteins, and result in tertiary structures that are not regarded as self by T cells. They elicit a type IV cell-mediated, delayed hypersensitivity, which is maximum forty-eight hours after exposure (see chapter 11).

This contact hypersensitivity is an epidermal phenomenon, whereas the well-known **tuberculin**-type hypersensitivity is mainly dermal in character. The principal antigen-presenting cell in contact dermatitis is the Langerhans cell, which comprises about 3 percent of cells in the epidermis. The characteristic skin reaction is due to the inflammatory response resulting from the release by activated T cells of various cytokines.

Anaphylaxis

This is a severe form of immediate hypersensitivity (type I), which results from the rapid release of histamine and other vascular permeability factors from mast cells and basophils. It occurs most commonly after a second dose of "foreign" serum, such as horse serum (source of antitoxin), and may result in rapid death. It also occurs after bee and wasp stings, intravenous administration of anesthetic agents, and eating some foods, particularly peanuts.

Human anaphylaxis is characterized by hypotension (low blood pressure), peripheral circulatory failure, urticaria (hives), and constriction of bronchi. Severe cases, referred to as anaphylactic shock, are sometimes fatal.

Anaphylactoid Reaction

This is an acute shock syndrome that resembles anaphylactic shock, but is not immunologically mediated. Various substances can cause it including endotoxin, anesthetic agents, and snake and bee venoms. This reaction results from the release of large amounts of histamine and other vascular permeability factors as a consequence of the direct effect of these agents on basophils.

Anaphylatoxins

These are the complement components C3a, C4a, and C5a that stimulate mast cell degranulation with release of histamine and other mediators of inflammation. When inoculated into animals they produce clinical signs similar to those of systemic anaphylaxis.

Atopy

This is the clinical manifestation of type I immediate hypersensitivity reactions including asthma, hay fever, allergic eczema, allergic rhinitis, and other allergies.

Genetic Effects

The genes of an individual may also have a role in allergy/anaphylaxis. Genes influence three basic features of the allergic response. The first is that of total IgE levels, which is associated with genes on chromosome 5q in humans. The second is that of allergen specific responses: these are linked with particular HLA **alleles**. For example, in studies of individuals sensitive to the AMBaV protein of ragweed, approximately 90 percent are the HLA-Dw2 genotype. The last feature is that of general hyper-responsiveness, which is also HLA-linked. Individuals that respond to a broad range of allergens are hyperresponsive. These individuals tended to have the genotypes HLA-B8 and HLA-Dw3, but not HLA-A1.

Diagnosis

The classical diagnostic test in atopy is the skin test, which involves injection of antigen into the skin. When positive, it leads to the release of mediators, increased vascular permeability, edema, and itching. It is known as the "wheal and flare" reaction. The results of this test correlate well with the frequently used radioallergosorbent test (RAST) on the patient's serum. This is a test for antigen-specific IgE in serum (see chapter 16).

Other diagnostic tests are the skin prick test, skin patch test (particularly for allergic contact dermatitis), and nasal provocation test. Some patients may be negative to an allergen with one test method but positive with another. Skin tests and RAST are often negative for food allergens and diagnosis is sought using an "elimination diet" followed by introduction of suspected foods.

Treatment

Most important is avoidance of the allergen completely or as much as is feasible. Allergists recommend measures to reduce exposure, such as banning a pet, using an air-conditioner, and removing dust collecting items.

Treatment mainly involves allergen immunotherapy (allergy injections) and/or administration of antihistamines. In the first approach small amounts of the allergen are injected into the skin in gradually increasing doses, until a maintenance level is achieved. This procedure, often referred to as desensitization, stimulates the body to produce neutralizing or blocking (IgG) antibodies that may reduce allergic reactions; the IgE level may also fall, possibly due to the induction of tolerance, a switch from a Th2 response to a Th1 response, or activation of T suppressor activities.

The antihistamines used to treat allergies are referred to as histamines$_1$ as they block the histamine$_1$ (H1) receptor. It is this receptor, when stimulated, that causes injury to target tissues.

Additionally, cromolyn sodium aids in stabilizing the cell membrane and preventing the influx of calcium ions that mediate degranulation. Theophylline acts on adenylate cyclase to increase intracellular cAMP levels and inhibit degranulation. Corticosteroids are used as anti-inflammatory agents against the late phase reaction. In severe anaphylaxis, epinephrine is administered, as it reverses the effects of histamine by relaxing smooth muscle and decreasing vascular permeability.

GLOSSARY

Allele—an alternative form of a gene situated at the corresponding site on a homologous chromosome.

cAMP—a derivative of ATP that occurs widely in animal cells as an intermediary messenger in many biochemical reactions induced by hormones.

Exocytosis—the release of secretory products from cell vesicles.

Nonapeptide—a peptide with nine amino acids.

Tuberculin—a protein extract obtained from the cells of *Mycobacterium tuberculosis*.

CHAPTER 11

Hypersensitivity Reactions, Part II: Cytotoxic/Cytologic Immune Complex, and Delayed-Type

Although the immune system is generally protective and beneficial, it can on occasion malfunction and give rise to immune disorders. Some of these disorders, which are discussed below, are due to hypersensitivity reactions. Four different types of hypersensitivity reactions have been described by Coombs and Gell, namely, types I, II, III, and IV. Hypersensitivity type I reactions are the allergy/anaphylaxis reactions that were described in chapter 10. This chapter describes the other three types of hypersensitivity reactions.

CYTOTOXIC/CYTOLYTIC REACTIONS

Type II hypersensitivity is observed when specific antibody binds antigen on a cell surface resulting in cytolysis, cell death from the activation of complement, or phagocytosis and destruction by macrophages and neutrophils.

Transfusion Reactions

These are the result of ABO incompatibility in blood transfusions. Based upon blood type, all individuals, except those who are AB, have preformed antibodies against other blood types, except O. For example, someone who is blood type O possesses circulating IgM antibodies against types A and B. The reason for these preformed antibodies is not known. However, with a transfusion of the wrong blood type an immediate reaction takes place within the bloodstream. IgM efficiently acti-vates the complement cascade, resulting in lysis of the RBCs. This in turn results in kidney damage due to the large quantity of cell mem-brane now present in circulation and the toxic effects due to release of the heme complex of hemoglobin.

Rh Incompatibility Reactions

This example of type II hypersensitivity is similar to what is observed with transfusion reactions. However, in this case the antigen is the Rh factor protein. This type of reaction is typically observed in mothers who are Rh- and a fetus that is Rh+. The sensitization of the mother typically occurs with the first offspring, when some red blood cells (RBCs) are released into the maternal circulation. The Rh factor is processed and presented to maternal T cells and stimulates an IgG response. With the conception of a second offspring, the anti-Rh IgG antibodies cross the placenta and react with fetal RBCs, leading to hemolysis within the fetus and eventually death of the fetus.

Treatment for Rh incompatibility typically involves giving the mother preformed anti-Rh antibodies immediately after the birth of the first child. These antibodies participate in the destruction of circulating fetal blood cells prior to the formation of the IgG response.

Autoimmune Reactions

These are the result of antibody production against self antigens, such as self RBCs. The reason for the stimulation of these antibodies is fre-quently unknown. In some instances it may be correlated with infec-tious disease. When the target is self RBCs the resulting condition leads to progressive autoimmune hemolytic anemia. Occasionally, these antibodies bind to the RBCs more efficiently at lower tempera-tures, as in individuals exposed to cold temperatures. They are thus referred to as cold agglutinins. For unknown reasons, most cold agglu-tinin anemia occurs in older people. Sometimes cold agglutinin ane-mia follows infection with *Mycoplasma pneumoniae*, the cause of pri-mary atypical pneumonia in humans. In this disease, the anemia is acute, of short duration, and thought to be due to response to a cross-reactive mycoplasmal antigen.

The kind of reactions just described can involve blood cells other than RBCs. If the antibody response is to platelets, the result is a **thrombocytopenia**, which leads to bleeding (purpura). Antibody responses to neutrophils and lymphocytes have been noted in individuals with systemic lupus erythematus, but the role of these antibodies in the pathogenesis of the disease is not clear.

Autoimmunity is discussed at length in chapter 12.

Drug-induced Reactions

In these reactions, drugs have complexed with cell surface proteins. The drug complexed with the cell surface protein becomes immunogenic and stimulates antibody production to the drug. When the drug is taken again, the drug again binds to the cell surface proteins and now makes these cells targets for antibody binding, phagocytosis, cytolysis, or activation and destruction by complement. Some examples of drugs that cause drug-induced reactions are the sedative sedormid, which binds to platelets leading to thrombocytopenia, and the antibiotic chloramphenicol, which may bind to white blood cells resulting in the disease **agranulocytosis**.

Antireceptor Antibody Diseases

In these diseases, binding of antibody to self receptors can lead to either cytolysis of cells or to continual stimulation of a cell via the receptor. Examples of these diseases are:

Myasthenia gravis. In this disorder, an antibody response is made against the acetylcholine receptors at the neuromuscular junction. The result is progressive muscle weakness resulting from increased receptor turnover and obstruction of the receptor by the IgG antibodies.

Grave's disease. The antibody response in this disease is to the thyroid stimulating hormone receptor in the thyroid. The antibodies bind the receptors and stimulate the thyroid cells to produce thyroid hormones resulting in hyperthyroidism.

Diagnosis

Diagnosis of type II hypersensitivity involves the detection of antibody or complement on target cells or tissue, or the detection of circulating antibodies to cell surface antigens, tissue antigens, receptor proteins, or an exogenous antigen. The most common assay for detection of antibody or complement associated with cells or tissue involves fluorescence microscopy (see chapter 16).

Treatment

The treatment is largely based upon the severity of the disease. It can range from nonsteroidal anti-inflammatory agents to high dose corticosteroid treatment and immunosuppressive drugs. In transfusion reactions, high doses of mannitol or furosemide are given to provide alternative targets for the antibody to maintain the integrity of as many RBCs as possible.

IMMUNE COMPLEX DISEASE

Immune complexes form when antibody molecules combine with corresponding antigens. The immune complex may be soluble and small, particularly in antigen excess, or large and precipitate at optimal proportions of antigen and antibody.

The large complexes are taken up by the liver and spleen and broken down by macrophages and other phagocytes through the interaction of the Fc portion of the antibody with complement and cell-surface receptors. However, these complexes sometimes persist and deposit in various tissues and organs resulting in immunopathologic changes.

The reaction responsible for immune complex disease is referred to as type III hypersensitivity and has three primary causes. The first is persistent infection, which typically results in damage to the kidney; the second is autoimmunity, which typically results in damage to the kidney, joints, arteries, and skin; and the third, chronic inhalation of antigen such as mold, plant, or animal antigens, which results in immune complexes in the lungs.

Mechanisms of Type III Hypersensitivity

The basic mechanisms of type III hypersensitivity are those that trigger inflammatory responses. In one mechanism, the immune complexes interact with complement, which releases C3a and C5a. In turn, these mediators stimulate cells to release vasoactive peptides such as histamine and chemotactic factors for basophils, eosinophils, and neutrophils.

Alternatively, macrophages can be stimulated by the complexes to release cytokines, particularly TNFα and IL-1, which are important in the inflammatory response. Immune complexes may also directly stimulate basophils and platelets by binding the Fc receptors of the cells and stimulating the release of vasoactive amines, which cause increased vascular permeability.

In many instances, the immune complexes deposit on blood vessel walls by a process called immune adherence. This causes platelets to aggregate at the site, forming **microthrombi**. Polymorphs attempt to engulf the immune complexes but cannot as they are adhered to the blood vessel wall. The lysosomal enzymes deposited at the site by polymorphs lead to endothelial damage (see fig. 11.1).

Some examples of type III hypersensitivity are described below.

Serum Sickness

The earliest disease found to be due to type III hypersensitivity is serum sickness. It can occur after the injection of a large amount of soluble foreign antigen, for instance, horse serum containing antitoxin used in treatment and prophylaxis of several diseases. Serum sickness is characterized by fever, swollen lymph nodes, urticaria, joint swellings, and sometimes renal lesions. The clinical signs are due to the localization of soluble immune complexes, which are continuously formed in the presence of excess antigen. They are formed faster than phagocytes can remove them.

Before the cause of serum sickness was known, its resemblance to what was called the Arthus reaction was noted early in this century.

Arthus Reaction

The Arthus reaction was first observed in rabbits. It is manifested by a local inflammatory reaction in the skin that occurs after adminis-

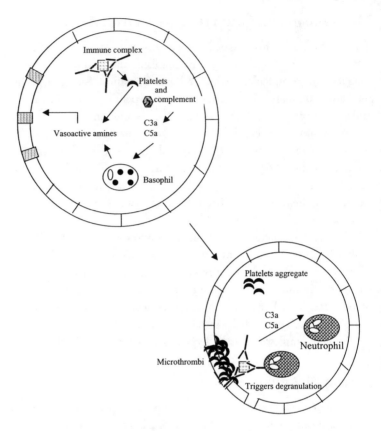

Figure 11.1. The effects of deposition of immune complexes in blood vessel walls

tration of antigen to an animal that already has precipitating antibodies to that antigen. The local edematous, inflammatory reaction follows the blockage of capillaries in the skin by small, soluble antigen-antibody complexes and leukocytes.

Small complexes may remain in circulation and in the presence of excess antigen they may penetrate the vascular lining of certain small blood vessels down to the basement membrane. The first component of complement, C1q, binds to the Fc portion of the complexed antibody and the complement cascade follows. Breakdown products of C3 and C5 interact with mast cells, polymorphs, and other cells to produce the vascular damage that is characteristic of immune complex disease. This kind of general reaction is referred to as type III immune complex hypersensitivity. Damage ensues from prolonged exposure to antigen and the continuous elicitation of antibody.

The cells lining many small vessels in an organ or tissue may be damaged. The inflammation may be chronic with the proliferation of new blood vessels and the replacement of damaged tissue with fibrous tissue.

A component of type III hypersensitivity is involved in a number of infectious diseases. The following are important human immune complex diseases:

Rheumatic Fever. This immune complex disease follows an infection with group A streptococci resulting in inflammation and damage to heart, joints, and kidneys. The cause is antigens of the streptococci that are cross-reactive with antigens of human heart muscle, cartilage, and glomerular basement membrane. These cross-reactive antibodies activate the complement cascade and stimulate the accumulation of neutrophils at the site, which become activated and release lysosomal enzymes, all of which serve to cause cell damage at the site.

Immune complex glomerulonephritis. In this disease, which has a number of causes, immune complexes accumulate in tubules and glomeruli of the kidneys. The inflammatory process and consequent tissue injury leads to renal dysfunction.

Farmer's Lung. This is a local immune complex occupational disease that results from the continual inhalation of antigen (moldy hay). When a sensitized individual is exposed to moldy hay, symptoms of severe respiratory distress appear within six to eight hours of exposure. The sensitized individual had an IgG response to the spores of thermophilic actinomycetes growing on the spoiled hay. Inhalation of the bacterial spores results in a response that resembles the Arthus reaction. Immune complexes form within the alveoli of the lung and the seriousness of the respiratory disease depends upon the severity and duration of the inflammatory reaction. Symptoms include fever, breathlessness in mild cases, and respiratory distress in severe cases and repeated exposures. Similar diseases are observed with occupations in which there is massive, chronic exposure to potentially antigenic material.

Type III Hypersensitivity in Autoimmune Disease

Immune complex disease may be responsible for chronic autoimmune disease (see chapter 12). In such diseases, self antigens are involved rather than foreign ones. Autoimmune diseases in which type III hypersensitivity is involved include rheumatoid arthritis and **Goodpasture's syndrome**.

Diagnosis

Some immune complexes can be precipitated by polyethylene glycol and assays are based on this property. As the complexes contain Ig they react with anti-Ig antibodies. Assays are available to measure Cq1, and C3 can be detected with anti-C3 antibody. Because not all immune complexes fix complement, other procedures may be necessary. The examination of biopsies for immune complexes may be indicated.

Treatment

Treatment is mainly symptomatic and varies with the particular immune complex disease.

TYPE IV DELAYED-TYPE HYPERSENSITIVITY

In contrast with the other types of hypersensitivities, type IV delayed-type hypersensitivity (DTH) is mediated primarily by a few antigen-specific T cells. These few T cells, upon exposure to antigen, release cytokines and chemokines that stimulate the recruitment of mononuclear cells to the site. These recruited mononuclear cells are responsible for the hypersensitivity reaction, a nonspecific response.

Delayed-type hypersensitivity reactions are stimulated by a variety of antigens including allografts (foreign tissue), intracellular parasites (viruses, mycobacteria, fungi), soluble proteins, and chemicals capable of penetrating the skin and binding to body proteins.

The DTH response was originally observed by Koch in 1890 when he noted that people with tuberculosis (*Mycobacterium tuberculosis*) responded to intradermal mycobacterial lysates within twenty-four to forty-eight hours. This positive response was characterized by both erythema (redness) and induration (thickening). These reactions rarely lead to necrosis and resolve slowly.

Mechanism of DTH

There are two stages in the mechanism of DTH: the sensitization stage and the elicitation stage.

THE SENSITIZATION STAGE

The sensitization stage lasts approximately two weeks and is initiated by antigen processing and presentation by an APC. This APC then interacts with a CD4+ Th1 cell (Td), which responds by secreting IL-2, IFNγ, and IL-12. IL-2 and IFNγ recruit macrophages to the area. IL-12 suppresses Th2 responses, allowing expansion of the Th1 response. The Th1 response involves cellular proliferation of T cells and secretion of more IL-2 and IFNγ for the recruitment of more macrophages.

THE ELICITATION STAGE

The elicitation stage begins with a reexposure to the antigen and results in the characteristic DTH response. One of the expanded Td cells interacts with an APC that has processed and presented the antigen with this second exposure. This time, the interaction results in the release of IL-2 (proliferation and activation of T cells), IFNγ (activates macrophages), TNFβ (cytotoxic), and macrophage chemotactic factor (MCF). All of these mediators attract and activate macrophages, stimulating the release of more cytokines and increasing the capacity of the macrophages to phagocytize and destroy. The consequences of this response are activation of macrophages, increased phagocytosis and release of lysosomal enzymes, and products of the respiratory burst (peroxide and super oxide radicals). If the antigen is readily removed by this process, the lesion will resolve slowly with little or no tissue damage. However, if the antigen is protected and persistent, such as with **schistosome** eggs or mycobacterial infections, the response is chronic. More and more macrophages accumulate at the site leading to the formation of granulomas, which displace the normal tissue eventually leading to caseous necrosis. The disease manifestations are not due to the pathogens themselves, but rather to the host's attempt to isolate and remove the pathogen or at least render it harmless.

In viral diseases such as smallpox, herpes, and measles, the characteristic rashes produced are in part the result of the DTH response toward the viral antigens. Further destruction of cells associated with these infections is the result of cytotoxic activity on epithelial cells infected with virus.

Variations of DTH

CONTACT SENSITIVITY

The target organ in contact sensitivity is the skin and the response is to a sensitizing substance, such as the poison ivy oil urushiol, which is secreted by the leaves of the plant. The antigen presenting cells (APCs) are the Langerhans cells in the epithelium and the DTH is stimulated by reexposure to the antigen. Also part of the DTH in this instance is the formation of blisters that result from a separation of the epidermal cells and intracellular edema of the spongy layer of the skin.

ALLOGRAFT REJECTION

This is an acute rejection due to a cell-mediated response and results from a mismatch of tissues (see chapter 14).

CUTANEOUS BASOPHIL HYPERSENSITIVITY

Cutaneous basophil hypersensitivity (CBH) has been observed in patients following repeated intranasal administration of antigen. There is delayed onset of this response, which consists of erythema with no observable induration. The primary cell type found at these sites is basophils. The response is T cell mediated, but the mechanism involved is currently unknown. Additionally, CBH has been noted in cases of contact dermatitis, rejection of kidney grafts, and some forms of conjunctivitis.

In guinea pigs, CBH has been observed at tick bite sites. Presumably, the basophils can mediate the death and release of the tick via the release of basophilic granules. This evidence suggests that CBH has a role in immunity to some external parasites.

Diagnosis

The patch test is commonly used for the diagnosis of DTH. In this procedure antigen is applied to the skin. The area is observed at forty-eight to seventy-two hours for signs of erythema and induration, which indicate that the patient is sensitive to that particular antigen. A variation of this method is the patch test for antigens other than tuberculin.

Treatment

If antigen can be removed, the DTH will resolve within days to weeks with little or no intervention required. If the antigen is persistent, corticosteroid treatment is indicated.

GLOSSARY

Agranulocytosis—a fall in the number of circulating neutrophils resulting from the depression of myelopoiesis (production of bone marrow cells).

Goodpasture's syndrome—this disease is due to a proliferative glomerulonephritis and the principal symptom is the coughing of blood (hemoptysis).

Microthrombi—small thrombi. A thrombus is an aggregation of blood elements that can cause vascular obstruction at the point of formation.

Schistosome—blood nematodes or flukes that cause schistomiasis; a severe disease occurring mainly in Africa, Asia, and South America.

Thrombocytopenia—a decrease in the number of blood platelets.

CHAPTER 12

Autoimmunity

Autoimmunity is humoral or cell-mediated immunity to antigens of the body's own tissues. Reactions between antibody or T cells and autoantigen ("self" antigens) can lead to tissue damage, which, if sufficient, is referred to as autoimmune disease. More than forty autoimmune diseases have been identified. Some of the better known ones are type I diabetes, rheumatoid arthritis, systemic lupus erythematosus, pernicious anemia, multiple sclerosis, Hashimoto's disease (hypothyroidism), and myasthenia gravis. The mechanism involved and the location of the effects in some important autoimmune diseases are given in table 12.1.

Autoimmune diseases comprise two major categories, organ specific and nonorgan specific disorders. One autoantigen may be involved as in Hashimoto's disease, an organ specific (thyroid) disorder, or a number of autoantigens as in systemic lupus erythematosus, a nonspecific organ (various tissues) disease (see table 12.1).

DEVELOPMENT

T and B cells destined to react with self antigens are eliminated (clonal deletion) or anergized (clonal anergy or clonal paralysis) during the process of lymphocyte maturation (see immunological tolerance in chapter 7 for details). Unfortunately in some individuals, the anergized T cells and B cells become reactivated. These self-reactive clones, if sufficiently active, may lead to autoimmune disease. As stated above these disorders may involve a humoral or cell-mediated immune response to various self antigens.

The inducing antigens associated with well-characterized, naturally occurring, autoimmune diseases are not known. However, the incidence of particular types of autoimmune disease has been correlated with specific HLA antigens. The presence of these HLA antigens does

Table 12.1. Some Human Autoimmune Diseases

Disease	Target tissue*
Diseases targeting a restricted range of tissues:	
Addison's disease	Adrenal glands
Autoimmune hemolytic anemia	Erythrocytes
Autoimmune hepatitis	Liver
Autoimmune nephritis	Kidney
Autoimmune (Hashimoto's) thyroiditis	Thyroid
Crohn's disease	Intestine
Diabetes (insulin-dependent)	Pancreas
Graves' disease	Thyroid
Goodpasture's syndrome	Kidney
Multiple sclerosis	Nervous system
Myasthenia gravis	Thymus
Pemphigus	Skin
Diseases targeting a wide range of tissues:	
Rheumatoid arthritis	
Scleroderma	
Sjögren's syndrome	
Systemic lupus erythematosus	

*Antibodies are produced against a constituent or constituents of a tissue, e.g., the basement membrane of kidney glomeruli in Goodpasture's syndrome.

not mean that an individual will necessarily develop autoimmune disease, as disease progression is multifactorial involving many genes in combination with environmental factors.

ROLE OF HEREDITY

An inherited tendency to develop certain of these disorders has long been suspected. There is now considerable evidence that heredity is an important influence in determining the incidence and type of autoimmune disease. It is also recognized that such factors as hormone levels and infection by certain bacteria and viruses may lead to autoimmune disease. Most of the autoimmune diseases studied show an association with HLA (see chapter 6) specificity.

The pattern of inheritance for autoimmune diseases is very complex and is thought to involve several genes. For example, in the mouse model, at least fourteen genes are associated with the development of type I diabetes mellitus. The counterparts of these genes in the human disease are currently unidentified.

Some examples in humans of HLA genes associated with particular autoimmune diseases include rheumatoid arthritis—HLA-DR1 and major subtypes of HLA-DR4; organ specific types—HLA-DR3 is common; Hashimoto's thyroiditis—HLA-DR5; and type I diabetes—HLA-DQ2/8 heterozygotes.

ENVIRONMENT

The role of the environment in the onset of autoimmunity is that of the "trigger." For example, autoreactive T and B cells to sequestered antigens are typically harmless as the antigens are never exposed to immune cells. These antigens include the proteins of the lens and uvea of the eye and spermatozoal antigens. However, if these antigens are introduced into the circulation as the result of trauma to the eye, for example, an autoimmune response will occur. Unfortunately, this does not explain the immune responses of the many autoimmune diseases currently identified. There are three mechanisms of control that are thought to be compromised and result in autoimmunity. They are described below.

Absence of Th cells

At low doses of antigen, tolerance is typically induced in T cells. Even though autoreactive B cells may be present in circulation, they do not present a problem because no T helper cells are available to augment the response.

Bypasses of control mechanism: New or altered carrier proteins activate Th cells and allow progression of the response. Nonspecific polyclonal activation, as observed with adjuvants and bacterial LPS, nonspecifically activates autoreactive B cell clones. The trigger in this instance is thought to be viral infections or certain drug therapies. For example, in some bacterial infections cross-reactive antigens are produced by group A streptococci that affect heart muscle. Infection with the Epstein-Barr virus or the presence of bacterial LPS nonspecifically mediates polyclonal activation, which includes potential autoreactive B cell clones.

Control by T Suppressor Activity

In the mouse model, when T suppressor activity is compromised by irradiation, there is an increased, quicker, and more severe incidence of autoimmune diseases.

Lack of MHC Class II Molecules on Target Cells

In order to respond to antigen, CD4+ T cells need the antigen to be presented in the context of the MHC class II molecule. Some antigens will only be presented by MHC class I molecules, but not MHC class II molecules. When this happens, no T help can be available to those antigens.

Bypasses of control mechanism: Some cells can be induced to express MHC class II molecules by exposure to interferon (IFN)γ and other cytokines that are concomitantly activated by the cytokines and become APCs. In some instances autoantigens are now presented in the context of MHC class II molecules.

EXAMPLES OF AUTOIMMUNE DISEASES

Some important autoimmune diseases with their target tissues and associated hypersensitivity states are listed in table 12.1.

Antibody Mediated

Autoimmune hemolytic anemia. Antibodies against self-RBCs (see type II hypersensitivity in chapter 11).

Myasthenia gravis. Antibodies against acetylcholine receptors at neuromuscular junctions (see type II hypersensitivity in chapter 11).

Graves disease. Antibodies against thyroid stimulating hormone receptor (see type II hypersensitivity in chapter 11).

Immune-Complex Mediated

Systemic lupus erythematosus. This disorder is characterized by a distinctive rash on the cheeks that occurs early in the progression of the disease. The autoimmune response has many target organs and causes fever, joint pain, and damage to the central nervous system, heart, and kidneys. The cause of the autoimmune response is unknown.

The most characteristic phenomenon associated with this disorder is the production of antibodies against nuclear antigens: double-stranded DNA, single-stranded DNA, and histone proteins. The best correlation of the disease, and significant in diagnosis, is the production of antibodies against double-stranded DNA.

T-cell Mediated

Multiple sclerosis. This disorder is characterized by the demyelinization of tissues of the central nervous system. Lesions associated with the disorder are cellular and similar to those observed with DTH. The cause of this autoimmune disorder is unknown.

Type I diabetes mellitus. This insulin-dependent form of diabetes is the result of chronic inflammatory destruction of the beta-islet cells of the pancreas by lymphocytes.

Hashimoto's thyroiditis. This T-cell mediated autoimmune response results in goiter formation or hypothyroidism. There is no known cause, and although the response is primarily T-cell mediated, antibody may contribute to the progression of the disease. As in multiple sclerosis, DTH-type lesions are observed.

T-cell and Antibody Mediated

Rheumatoid arthritis. This condition is the result of chronic inflammation of the joint synovium, eventually leading to destruction of cartilage and bone. The synovial membrane becomes highly cellular, to the point of resembling lymphoid tissue, all of which contributes to erosion of the joint. Found in these lymphoid areas are antigen-antibody complexes, complement, neutrophils, T cells, activated macrophages, and NK cells. Concomitantly there is a plethora of cytokines, enzymes, and other mediators present in these areas. Together, these cells and mediators contribute to the destruction of cartilage and damage to the joint ensues.

Deficiency in Complement Components

There has been some correlation with deficiencies in early complement components (C1, C4, C2) and development of autoimmune diseases, such as systemic lupus erythematosus.

DIAGNOSIS

A variety of immunological tests are used to detect the autoantibodies involved in autoimmune diseases. For example, immunofluorescence and precipitin tests (see chapter 16 for these procedures) are used to detect autoantibodies to thyroglobin in Hashimoto's disease. An agglutination test is used to detect antibodies to sperm in autoimmune male infertility. Biopsy and indirect immunofluorescence assay are used to detect mitochondrial antibody in autoimmune hepatitis (biliary cirrhosis). A polyethylene glycol assay (precipitation of immune complexes) and immunofluorescence staining (biopsy) are used for the detection of immune complexes in systemic lupus erythematosus and other nonorgan-specific autoimmune diseases. Another procedure for circulating complexes employs a radioimmunoassay for detection of complement C1q. Some of the serologic tests and procedures referred to above are described in chapter 16.

Diagnosis is based on the results of these tests along with other laboratory data and clinical findings. The presence of autoantibodies has predictive value in that they may be present for relatively long periods before overt disease.

TREATMENT

Systemic lupus erythematosus, which involves several autoantigens in a number of tissues, can be controlled only by immunosuppressive therapy. Such organ-specific disorders as type I diabetes and Hashimoto's disease can be controlled with insulin and thyroxin, respectively. The treatment for many of the autoimmune diseases is mainly symptomatic.

CHAPTER 13

Immunodeficiencies

The immune system is remarkably complex and its function depends upon the interaction of many factors. Although it performs efficiently in most individuals, it is subject to a variety of defects that can, albeit infrequently, impair its normal function. Immunodeficiencies may result from acquired or genetic defects.

Immunodeficiencies are classified as primary (the direct result of genetic or acquired immunodeficiency) or secondary (the indirect result of genetic or acquired immunodeficiency, such as disease). Some of the more important and familiar immunodeficiencies are summarized below.

PRIMARY IMMUNODEFICIENCIES

Stem cells

• *X-linked severe combined immunodeficiency.*
Stem cells are absent and thus are not in lymphoid tissue.
Example: Swiss type gammaglobulinemia.
No humoral or cell-mediated immunity.
Treatment: bone marrow transplant.

T lymphocyte

• *Absence of thymus and parathyroids; maldevelopment of the third and fourth pharyngeal pouch derivatives.*
Di George syndrome: no T lymphocytes.
Nezelof syndrome: Similar to Di George syndrome, but parathyroids are normal.
• *Purine nucleoside phosphorylase (PNP) deficiency.*
An **autosomal** recessive defect in which toxic metabolites accumulate in T cells resulting in a deficiency in cell-mediated immunity.
Treatment: thymus transplant.

B lymphocyte

• *X-linked agammaglobulinemia or hypogammaglobulinemia.*
Absence of germinal centers in lymph nodes and spleen.
Failure of B cells to differentiate into plasma cells.
Inability to make one class of immunoglobulin, usually IgA, but occasionally IgG or IgM. No humoral immunity.
Example: Bruton type hypoglobulinemia.
Response to chemotaxis may be impaired.
Treatment: administration of immunoglobulin.

Granulocytes

• *Reduced numbers of neutrophils.*
Example: infantile agranulocytosis.
• *Chronic granulomatous disease* (CGD).
Due to a defect in the oxidative microbicidal function of neutrophils leading to chronic bacterial or fungal infection.
Result: Recurring suppurative inflammation of lymph nodes; visceral abscesses and pulmonary granulomas.
• *Chediak-Higashi syndrome.*
An autosomal recessive disease of children making them particularly susceptible to pyogenic (pus producing) bacterial infections. Failure of neutrophils to digest ingested bacteria. Lysosomal granules are abnormally large; neutrophils are deficient in killing and digesting bacteria.
Treatment: blood transfusion; bone marrow transplant.

Defects Involving More Than One Type of Cell

• *Reticular dysgenesis* (Ret. dys.). This involves a complete deficiency of stem cells. Those affected do not survive more than a few days after birth.
• *Ataxia telangectasia* (Atax. tel.). This autosomal immunodeficiency syndrome is seen in children with thymic hypoplasia and B and T cell defects. It results in oculocutaneous telangectasia (dilation of capillaries), cerebellar ataxia, and progressive dementia.
• *Severe combined immunodeficiency* (SCID). This is a rare immunodeficiency of infants that is characterized by early infections and diar-

rhea. Both cell-mediated (T cells) immunity and humoral (B cells) immunity are defective. Various forms of SCID occur. One form is X-linked in which there is a complete absence of T cells. There is an autosomal recessive form in which there is a deficiency of the enzyme adenosine deaminase (also known as ADA deficiency).

Treatment: blood transfusions; bone marrow transplant; gene therapy.

• *Wiskott-Aldrich syndrome* (Wisk. Ald.). The antibody response to polysaccharide antigens is defective as is the cell-mediated immune response. The cause of this X-linked deficiency may be a deficient expression of CD4 on leukocytes. There is combined deficiency in both T and B cell functioning. There is a low blood platelet count, eczema, a high incidence of tumors and recurrent infections.

Treatment: splenectomy, continuous antibiotics, intravenous immunoglobulin, bone marrow transplant.

SECONDARY DEFICIENCIES

Deficiencies in immune mechanisms can be acquired from or associated with the following:

• *Age*. The immune response tends to be weaker in old age and infancy (up to three to four months). Passively transferred maternal antibodies augment immunity in infancy.

• *Tumors*. **Hodgkin's disease**, **multiple myeloma**, leukemia, and **lymphosarcoma** are often associated with immune deficiencies.

• *Excessive loss of protein*. This secondary immunodeficiency is the result of the loss of serum proteins (including antibodies) via the kidney (renal damage), skin (severe burns or dermatitis), or gastrointestinal tract (**enteropathy**). Often coupled with serum protein loss through the gastrointestinal tract, lymphocytes may also be lost contributing to **lymphopenia** and cellular immunodeficiency. Affected individuals are susceptible to gram-positive bacterial infections.

• *Malnutrition*: Reduces antibody production and in severe cases T cell production. Protein, caloric intake, vitamins, and certain minerals are important. Deficiencies associated with decreased antibody production and T cell function are as described previously.

• *Infections*: A number of infections can cause immunosuppression. Most notable is acquired immune deficiency syndrome (AIDS), which mainly involves infection of CD4+ T cells (see chapter 17). In measles, T cells are likely to be suppressed, leading to a reduction in cell-mediated responses. The same is true for infections with other viruses, such as rubella, cytomegalovirus, infectious mononucleosis, acute bacterial diseases, severe mycobacterial infections, and fungal diseases.

GLOSSARY

Autosome—a chromosome other than a sex chromosome.

Enteropathy—a disease of the intestinal tract.

Hodgkin's disease—a lymphoma (a neoplasm) characterized by the progressive enlargement of the liver, spleen, and lymph nodes. Normal lymphoid cells are replaced by neoplastic, multinucleate giant cells.

Lymphopenia—a reduced lymphocyte count.

Lymphosarcoma—a malignant lymphoma with a tendency to metastasize (spread).

Multiple myeloma—a neoplasm of the bone marrow characterized by the presence of numerous myelomas in various bones. The cells involved in myelomas may be any one of the bone marrow cells.

CHAPTER 14

Transplantation and Graft Rejection

Transplantation or grafting involves introducing an organ or tissue to an individual. This can be accomplished successfully between identical (syngeneic) twins, but rejection takes place between nonsyngeneic humans. This (rejection) is due to the fact that most cells bear major histocompatibility complex (MHC) antigens that vary greatly between people (see chapter 6). The likelihood that many of these antigens are the same for any two unrelated humans is minimal. The immune system operates by detecting foreign MHC proteins on transplanted cells and reacting strongly to them. This constitutes rejection and is the basic problem in transplantation.

REJECTION

Initially "altered self" class II MHC antigens are recognized by T-helper cells. Antigen-presenting cells trigger B cells, macrophages, and cytotoxic T cells into action along with complement. The action initiated and the results vary with the target cells. The following are involved in rejection:

• Antibody, along with complement, destroys cells that are free in blood and lymph.
• T cells attach to and can lyse cells within solid tissues directly.
• Macrophages are active against foreign tissue in type IV delayed-type hypersensitivity.
• Vascular endothelium is attacked initiating type III complex-mediated hypersensitivity.

The body's response to various organs and tissues varies as indicated:

Bone marrow. This tissue is strongly rejected and requires potent immunosuppression.

Cartilage and cornea. Being nonvascular and lacking MHC antigens, they survive. This is true as long as the antigens remain sequestered during the transplant procedure.

Endocrine glands. They survive well if the small number of cells with class II antigens are removed prior to transplantation.

Heart. Although heart transplants are not as successful as kidney transplants, most recipients live at least five years.

Kidney. The success of renal transplants has greatly increased in recent years and approaches 70 percent. Rejection is described as follows: immediate—due to mismatch or the presence of antibodies to MHC antigens; acute—taking weeks to months as a result of the host's immune response; chronic—involves months to years due to the development of immune complexes.

Liver. Generally, transplants are not strongly rejected.

Skin. Grafting is not a problem when one's own skin (autograft) is used. Skin allografts are used to provide temporary cover in the case of burns.

Fetus. The normal fetus is an allograft but for reasons not fully understood it is not rejected.

Most of the organs and tissues not mentioned above, such as lungs, pancreas, and spleen, have had low transplant success.

Clinical Features of Allograft Rejection

Allograft refers to a graft exchanged between two genetically dissimilar individuals of the same species.

HYPERACUTE REJECTION

This occurs within a few minutes to a few hours after transplantation. Destruction is mediated by preformed antibodies, such as ABO incompatibility antibodies, which rapidly activate complement and the activation and deposition of platelets. These combined reactions lead to local swelling and hemorrhage that ultimately decrease blood flow through the transplanted organ. Cell-mediated responses are not observed with this type of rejection. There is no treatment for this type of rejection.

ACUTE REJECTION

This type of allograft rejection is cell-mediated and is typically caused by the mismatching of tissues. In contrast with hyperacute rejections, acute reactions occur within a few days to two weeks following the transplantation. This type of rejection can be reduced by immunosuppressive therapy.

CHRONIC REJECTION

This type of allograft reaction is mediated by cellular and humoral responses. Chronic rejection reaction occurs months following transplantation. There is no treatment for this type of rejection.

Graft Versus Host Reactions

These are the result of the transfer of immunocompetent lymphocytes from the donor to the recipient. The reaction involves the response of the donor lymphocytes against recipient tissues. This is a problem when the transfer is to an immunocompromised host, as in bone marrow transplants, as the recipient cannot reject the transplanted cells. The donor lymphocytes recruit recipient inflammatory cells via cytokines and other mediators, resulting in tissue damage.

Immunosuppression

The reaction to foreign cells is variable. The antigens on some cells react more strongly than those on other cells. As mentioned above, liver cells are not strongly rejected. In order to reduce rejection responses, the following treatments are used for immunosuppression:

Cyclosporin A. This compound isolated from a soilborne fungus is the most potent immunosuppressant available. It is much less toxic and more inhibitory of organ rejection than any previous immunodepressants. Previous drugs had suppressed almost the entire immune system whereas cyclosporin A acts specifically to block the activation of T cells. Side effects include nausea, excessive hair growth, and renal toxicity.

FK-506. This drug, also isolated from a soil fungus, is as effective as cyclosporin A.

Cytotoxic drugs. These nonspecifically suppress lymphocyte division and are mainly used postoperatively.

Corticosteroids/Azathioprene. These are used postoperatively for their anti-inflammatory and nonspecific immunosuppressive effects.

Prednisone. This steroid has a nonspecific immunosuppressive action on both humoral and cell-mediated immunity.

Monoclonal antibodies to T cells. These are used to treat acute rejection.

Antilymphocyte globulin. This is used as a specific immunosuppressant against T lymphocytes.

Much current research is directed to the development of better procedures, drugs, and immunological products for transplantation.

Matching and Typing

For organ or tissue transplantation, MHC and ABO blood group antigens must be typed. Microtoxicity tests using B lymphocytes, monospecific antisera, and complement are employed for the MHC antigens. B lymphocytes carry class I and class II MHC antigens. The success of kidney transplants is attributed in part to the degree of match. The DR locus (one of three class II gene loci, see chapter 6) plays the most important role in tissue reaction. The best transplant results are obtained by matching the tissue at this locus. Compatibility is tested by the mixed lymphocyte reaction (see chapter 16).

Xenotransplantation

The great shortage in human donor organs has led to research into the possible use of organs from primates (concordant species) and nonprimates (discordant species). Transplants from animals are referred to as xenografts or xenotransplants. Currently there is much interest in pigs because they are more available than primates and there is less objection to their use. Porcine valves are already being used to replace human heart valves.

Efforts are being made to introduce human genes into pigs, which will result in their organs, such as heart and liver, being less foreign. Theoretically, genetically engineered pigs could provide hearts and other organs that produce no foreign antigens, only human ones. The recent success in cloning adult animals indicates that genetically identical animals including those with human genes will soon be readily produced.

A major drawback to the use of animal tissues and organs is the chance that they may harbor viruses that are pathogenic for humans. There has been an instance of a virus in pig cells crossing over and infecting human cells. Recently, Britain has placed a moratorium on the use of xenotransplants.

In addition to bone marrow (stem cells) transplants, cells taken from fetuses are being used to ameliorate Parkinson's disease, a form of diabetes, and some autoimmune disorders. When implanted, these cells are much less likely to be rejected than are whole organs.

CHAPTER 15

Vaccination and Immunization

The experimental foundation of immunology began with the epochal investigations of Jenner in 1796. He demonstrated that the infection of humans with cowpox virus induced protection against the deadly virus of smallpox. Prior to this, an Asian technique for immunization against smallpox was to expose uninfected individuals to the scab and fluids from smallpox lesions. This technique, called variolation, was introduced in England and the American colonies in 1721. However, protection was not always provided by this method and the presence of live virus sometimes led to the development of smallpox. As a consequence, variolation was abandoned. Jenner's method of immunization to prevent smallpox, which was used for many years, and Pasteur's brilliant development of a vaccine to prevent rabies, are among the most important in medicine (see Milestones in Immunology in chapter 1).

The development of effective vaccines against a wide range of diseases has resulted in an impressive decline in human mortality rates over the years. A signal achievement of vaccination was the final eradication of smallpox from the world in 1977. In addition to the saving of countless human lives, veterinary vaccines have greatly reduced the losses to infectious diseases of domestic animals.

NATURAL AND ARTIFICIAL IMMUNIZATION

When many infectious agents infect a host, they may produce an asymptomatic or subclinical infection, rather than one characterized by clinical signs. Such subclinical infection elicits natural immunity of varying duration to the particular infectious agent. This kind of immunity protects us from many infections, including hepatitis A, streptococcal infections, and the common cold.

In contrast to actively acquired immunity, there is immunity resulting from deliberate or artificial immunization, which includes vaccination. This involves exposing individuals to an altered infectious agent or a part thereof (active immunization) or providing the individual with specific antibodies (from an extraneous source) to an infectious agent for the purpose of passively protecting the individual from the particular agent (passive immunization).

ACTIVE IMMUNIZATION

Active immunization is usually referred to as vaccination. The word "vaccine" was introduced by Pasteur to commemorate Jenner's work with cowpox virus (vaccinia). Vaccine is a very general term that denotes all agents or constituents of agents used to induce specific immunity for the purpose of protecting against infectious disease.

Important considerations in the use of vaccines are:

- The immune system is not fully developed in the first months of life.
- Antibodies are passively transferred from the mother via the placenta (transplacental) and milk. This antibody can interfere with the immune response to a vaccine. For this reason the first vaccination is not usually given until the baby is six months of age, at which time passive antibody is no longer present. Exceptions to this rule are those vaccines that stimulate a humoral immune response to particular antigens, such as hepatitis B, which is given at birth. See table 15.1 for the recommended vaccination schedule in the United States.
- Premature babies have less passive antibody.
- The primary immune response is predominantly IgM, which is transient.
- The secondary response is IgG, which is long-lived.
- The anamnestic response is the strong secondary antibody response that occurs about seven days after the initial administration of antigen.
- Local and systemic immunity. Briefly, local immunity is mucosal and dependent generally on secretory IgA. In contrast, systemic immunity is dependent on circulating serum antibody. The oral, live polio vaccine elicits both local and systemic immunity whereas the inactivated polio vaccine induces only systemic immunity.

• Adjuvants are used to enhance the immune response. They act by retaining the immunogen at the injection site, as by a depot effect, thus delaying its release. The antigenic stimulation is prolonged and consequently increased. Salts of metals, such as those of aluminum, oil emulsions (Freund's adjuvants), and synthetic lipid vesicles (liposomes), are some of the adjuvants used.

• Active immunization may also elicit a cell-mediated immune response particularly if live microorganisms are administered.

VACCINES

A variety of vaccines is employed including the following:

Inactivated. These are vaccines in which the microorganisms have been killed by various means. They are safer than vaccines containing live

Table 15.1. Recommended Vaccination Schedule in the United States

Age	Vaccine
Birth	Hepatitis B
1–2 months	Hepatitis B
2 months	DTP*, injectable polio, Haemophilus influenzae type b polysaccharide
4 months	DTP*, injectable polio, Haemophilus influenzae type b polysaccharide
6 months	DTP*, Haemophilus influenzae type b polysaccharide
12 months	Chicken pox
15 months	MMR†, DRP*, oral polio
4–6 years	DTP*, oral polio
14–16 years (boosters every 10 years)	DT‡
18–24 years	MMR†
25–64	Measles, rubella
> 65 years	Influenza, pneumococcal disease

*DTP= diphtheria, tetanus, acellular pertussis
†MMR= measles, mumps, rubella
‡DT= tetanus with reduced quantity of diphtheria

agents but less immunogenic. Examples: cholera, polio, influenza, and whooping cough vaccines.

Live attenuated. The agents in these vaccines are nonpathogenic or have been weakened by various means, including genetic alteration (see below), so that they produce a mild, subclinical infection that results in strong protection. They are less safe than inactivated vaccines because they are live and may cause disease in immunocompromised individuals. Reversion to virulent state is a possibility. Examples: oral polio, measles, mumps, and yellow fever vaccines.

Toxoids. These are used to prevent diseases like tetanus and diphtheria that are caused by strong exotoxins. The toxin is modified or weakened in such a manner that its toxicity but not its capacity to immunize has been destroyed. Treatment of the toxin with formaldehyde is most often used.

Capsular polysaccharides. Vaccines consisting of these are used to prevent pneumococcal pneumonia and meningococcal infection.

Virus subunit vaccines. These are prepared by removing the nonessential components of the virus and leaving only the immunogenic protein.

Some of the widely used human vaccines are listed in table 15.2 along with indications and comments.

CURRENT AND NEW VACCINE DEVELOPMENT

The approaches to vaccine development are numerous and only several are mentioned below.

• Attenuation of disease agents by gene-segment reassortment or mutations. Using recombinant gene technologies, these agents are rendered "less virulent" by making specific errors in gene products that develop severe disease, while allowing the organism to survive long enough within the host in order to mount an adequate immune response.

• Anti-idiotype vaccines: Anti-idiotypic antibodies are made in a two-step process. First an antigen is introduced, to which an organism has an immune response. These antibodies are then used to immunize

Table 15.2. Types of Vaccines Used to Prevent Important Infectious Diseases of Humans

Disease	Type of Vaccine Used
Bacterial Diseases	
Diphtheria	Toxoid
Tetanus	Toxoid
Pertussis	Acellular fractions of *Bordetella pertussis*
Bacterial pneumonia	Purified polysaccharide from *Streptococcus pneumoniae*
Haemophilus influenzae meningitis	Conjugated vaccine (type b polysaccharide conjugated to a carrier protein)
Viral Diseases	
Measles	Attenuated virus
Mumps	Attenuated virus
Rubella	Attenuated virus
Polio	Injectable= inactivated virus Oral= attenuated virus
Influenza	Inactivated virus
Hepatitis B	Recombinant DNA vaccine or inactivated virus
Chicken pox (Varicella)	Attenuated virus

a second individual to which an immune response is made. Some of these antibodies have the antigenic characteristics of the original antigen (see fig. 15.1). These are called anti-idiotype antibodies. Thus far, anti-idiotype vaccines have been used only experimentally.

• DNA vaccines: In this approach the gene of the immunogen is introduced, for example, by a plasmid, to the genome of the host where it is responsible for producing the immunogen. The latter elicits antibodies that protect the host.

• Conjugate vaccines: The *Haemophilus influenzae* (a cause of bacterial meningitis in children) conjugate vaccine involves the conjugation of the immunogenic polysaccharide with a protein carrier. The immune response obtained with the conjugate product was much greater than with the polysaccharide alone.

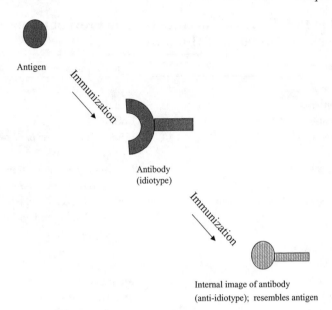

Figure 15.1. Generation of an anti-idiotypic antibody. Immunization with an antigen leads to the production of antibodies against the antigen (idiotype). Immunization with the idiotypic antibodies leads to the production of antibodies against the idiotypic antibody, some of which are similar to the original antigen (those directed against the Fab portion of the idiotypic antibody).

• Synthetic vaccines: In developing such products, attempts are made to synthesize pure microbial antigens, usually peptides or polypeptides, using recombinant and chemical techniques.

• Viral or bacterial carrier vaccines: These vaccines involve using recombinant gene techniques to place the genes of one or several pathogens in one carrier organism, either a virus or a bacterium. The carriers are a target of the immune response, in addition to the antigens that have been engineered to be expressed by the carrier. For example, *Salmonella typhimurium* could be a bacterial carrier expressing genes for influenza virus. Work on this type of vaccine is still in the experimental stage.

PASSIVE IMMUNIZATION

The transplacental passage of IgG from mother to fetus is a physiologic form of passive immunization. This transfer takes place during the last two months of gestation. Traces of this transplacental antibody may persist for as long as twelve months.

Passive immunization is generally used to provide temporary immunity to unimmunized individuals at high risk. Immune serum can be lifesaving when administered in cases of snake and spider bite, rabies exposure, botulism, and hepatitis B.

The products of human origin used for passive immunization comprise two main categories: standard immune serum globulin and special immune globulins. The former is from large groups of adult donors and the latter are all taken from individuals after exposure to particular diseases.

At one time, immune sera were produced solely in animals, usually horses, but because of the hypersensitivity (serum sickness) that sometimes developed, human serum of the two categories mentioned above is usually preferable. Tetanus, botulinus, and diphtheria antitoxins are prepared in horses.

CHAPTER 16

Immunodiagnostic Techniques

This chapter deals with the application of the principles of immunology to the diagnosis of infectious diseases. Some of the procedures described here have been adapted to convenient commercial test kits that are used widely by physicians and public-health related laboratories for the diagnosis of infectious diseases.

ANTIBODY DETECTION AND MEASUREMENT

Infection by many microbial pathogens elicits a specific antibody response. The detection and measurement of these antibodies are useful in the diagnosis of many infectious diseases. It is not always possible to isolate the causal pathogen in all infectious diseases.

In tests for antibody, a series of dilutions of serum with antigen are set up in order to determine the antibody titer (the highest dilution at which there is an antigen-antibody reaction) to a particular pathogen. To interpret the significance of antibody titers it is often helpful to test **"acute and convalescent" serum** samples, sometimes referred to as "paired" serum samples. Not all infections result in appreciable antibody response, for example, gonorrhea.

The various tests or assays for antibodies are carried out in numerous forms including tubes, microtiter plates with numerous small wells, glass slides, membranes, plates, and agar gels using pipettes to make dilutions and add reagents.

The principal immunodiagnostic techniques are described briefly below.

PROCEDURES

Agglutination Tests

This is the binding of particulate antigen by antibody resulting in an observable clumping or aggregation. An agglutination test in which the antigen is *Brucella* bacteria is used in the diagnosis of brucellosis (human undulant fever). Similar tests are used in the diagnosis of yersiniosis, leptospirosis, and tularemia. Whole parasites including leishmania, plasmodia, and *Toxoplasma gondii* are used in agglutination tests.

Antigens both soluble and particulate (e.g., some viruses) can be adsorbed to carrier red cells. When these coated red cells are mixed with specific antibody, hemagglutination takes place. This passive or indirect hemagglutination test is used for the diagnosis of a number of diseases. Some viruses agglutinate certain red cells directly and thus hemagglutination-inhibitions tests can be used to detect and measure antibodies.

PARTICLE AGGLUTINATION TESTS

Antigen can be bound to the surface of a carrier particle (e.g., latex). These coated particles are used in agglutination tests to detect antibody. Many systems using particle agglutination tests are available commercially for the diagnosis of a wide variety of bacterial, viral, fungal, and protozoal diseases.

Antibody can also be bound to particles and used to detect antigen in body fluids, for example, cryptococcal antigen in cerebrospinal fluid. Cryptococcosis is an important fungal disease of humans.

Precipitation Tests

These tests are based on the reaction between antibody and soluble antigen resulting in observable antigen-antibody complexes.

IMMUNODIFFUSION TEST/GEL DIFFUSION OR PRECIPITIN TEST/OUCHTERLONY DOUBLE DIFFUSION TEST

This is a precipitin test in which soluble antigen is placed in a well in an agar gel near a well containing antibody. The antigen and antibody diffuse toward one another and a specific reaction results in a visible precipitate within forty-eight hours (see fig. 16.1).

This procedure is used in the diagnosis of blastomycosis, histoplasmosis, coccidioidomycosis, and other fungal diseases.

Counterimmunoelectrophoresis (CIE)

In this procedure antigen or antibody is detected by a visible line or band of precipitation, which develops when the reactants in closely

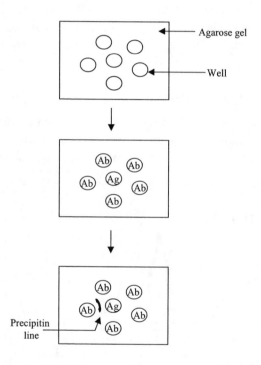

Figure 16.1. Double diffusion technique. Agarose gels are poured and allowed to solidify. A special cutting tool is used to cut the wells into the agarose on the pattern diagrammed above. Antigen (Ag) is added to the central well and test samples of the antibody (Ab) in the surrounding wells. (Conversely, antibody can be placed in the central well and antigen samples in the surrounding rings.) The antigen and antibody diffuse through the agarose. Where antigen-antibody reactions take place, a visible precipitin line forms. If there is no or extremely low levels of antigen-antibody complex formation, this precipitin line is not visible.

spaced wells, in a gel or on special paper, are moved toward one another by an electric current. The line of precipitation forms when the reactants meet at optimal proportions. This procedure is not widely used because it must be very carefully controlled.

ROCKET ELECTROPHORESIS

This technique is used to quantify antigen. As shown in figure 16.2, dilutions of antigen are placed in wells of a gel containing antibody to the particular antigen. With the passage of an electric current in the direction shown in the figure 16.2, lines of precipitation form in the shape of rockets. The height of the rockets is proportional to the amount of antigen in the well.

FLOCCULATION TESTS

The well-known VDRL (Venereal Disease Research Laboratory) test is used in the diagnosis of syphilis. The antigen (not spirochete derived) used is cardiolipin-lecithin coated cholesterol particles; the "antibody" is an anti-

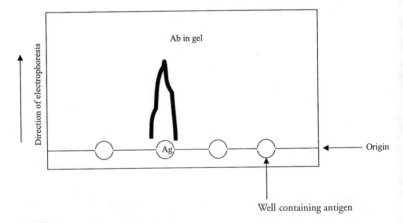

Figure 16.2. Rocket electrophoresis. An agarose gel is prepared containing a predetermined concentration of antibody (Ab). Wells are cut into the agarose once it has solidified and are filled with antigen. An electric current is then passed through the gel in the direction indicated by the diagram. Antigen-antibody complexes can be visualized as the antigen migrates through gel and appears in a rocket shape.

body-like protein called reagin, which occurs in individuals with syphilis. With positive reactions, macroscopically visible clumps are formed.

Neutralization Assays

These are tests in which antibody is measured by its capacity to neutralize the biological effects of an antigen often in the form of a virus or a bacterial toxin.

Virus neutralization tests determine the effect of dilutions of antibody on the infectivity of virus for cell cultures. These tests are time-consuming and technically demanding and for this reason they are usually performed in reference laboratories.

The ability of a serum to neutralize the erythrocyte-lysing capability of streptolysin O (a *Streptococcus pyogenes* toxin) is used to determine if there has been a previous streptococcal infection.

Complement Fixation (CF)

This rather complex test consists of two distinct systems: the first is the test system, and the second is the indicator system. The test is carried out as follows: The test serum is titered by doubling dilutions and a known amount of antigen is added to each well or tube. If antibody is present antigen-antibody complexes will form. Complement is added to the mixture and if complexes are present they will fix it. Red cells along with a subagglutinating amount of erythrocyte antibody are added to the mixture. If there is any complement present the red cells will be lysed. All aspects of this test must be carefully controlled if results are to be reliable.

Complement fixation tests have been largely supplanted by less-demanding procedures such as ELISA, particle agglutination, and indirect immunofluorescence. It is mainly used to detect antiviral and antifungal antibodies.

Enzyme-linked Immunosorbent Assay (ELISA)

This is the most important of several immunoassays. It is a procedure for the measurement of antibody or antigen. In measuring antibody, a known amount of antigen is adsorbed to the surface of wells, plastic tubes, beads, or other receptacle. Dilutions of the serum being tested are added to the antigen. After washing, an antiglobulin tagged with an enzyme (usually horseradish peroxidase or alkaline phosphatase) is added. If one is testing a human serum, a human **antiglobulin** is used. After washing, the substrate for the enzyme is added. The action of the enzyme on the substrate results in a detectable color, which can be measured spectrophotometrically. The amount of color produced is proportional to the amount of antibody present (see fig. 16.3).

The antigen can be measured conversely by applying specific antibody to the surface of the wells, tubes, beads, and such. The ELISA is remarkably sensitive.

Capture ELISA

This too is a powerful technique and is used when one wishes to detect antigen levels or cytokine levels in blood. In this procedure, a mono-

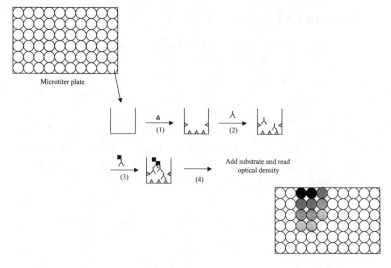

Figure 16.3. ELISA. (1) Wells of a microtiter plate are coated with antigen at a specific concentration. (2) Serum samples (antibody) are added to the different wells. (3) The enzyme-linked antibody is then added, which binds to the bound antibodies of the serum. (4) The substrate for the enzyme is then added. This results in a detectable change in color or fluorescence, which can then be measured spectrophotometrically.

clonal antibody is used to coat the microtiter plate. The serum sample is added to the wells. If viral antigens or certain cytokines are present in the sample, they will bind with the antibodies coated on the plate. After washing, a second monoclonal antibody is added to the same antigen that has been conjugated with an enzyme. The remainder of the assay is the same as for the ELISA (see fig. 16.4).

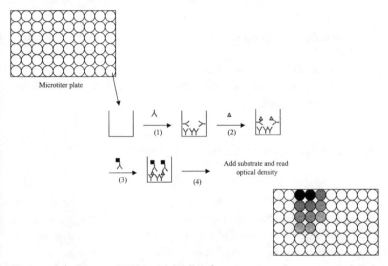

Figure 16.4. Capture ELISA. (1) Wells of a microtiter plate are coated with antibody at a specific concentration. (2) Serum samples (antigen) are added to the different wells. (3) The enzyme-linked antibody is then added, which binds to the bound antigen from the serum. (4) The substrate for the enzyme is then added. This results in a detectable change in color or fluorescence, which can then be measured.

Direct and Indirect Fluorescent Antibody Staining

These procedures are used widely to identify pathogenic microorganisms. A number of commercial diagnostic kits are available using these fluorescent techniques.

Direct method. **Fluorescein**-tagged antibody (specific for the antigen being sought) is applied to an antigen (can be a microorganism) fixed on a slide (can be a smear or tissue section). After reaction the excess antibody is washed off and the slide is examined under an ultraviolet (UV) microscope. If there has been an antigen-antibody reaction it will be seen as apple-green areas of fluorescence.

Indirect method. A specific antibody (unlabeled) is applied to the antigen smear and given time to react. After washing, a fluorescein-tagged antiglobulin specific for the unlabeled globulin is added. The antiglobulin by its binding or lack thereof will indicate whether or not there was antigen-antibody reaction. The presence of fluorescein-tagged antiglobulin will appear under UV light as apple-green fluorescence.

Horseradish peroxidase, alkaline phosphatase, and other enzymes can also be conjugated to specific antibodies for use in stains to detect various microorganisms.

INDIRECT IMMUNOFLUORESCENCE ASSAY

In this procedure antigen is adsorbed to plastic tubes, wells, or other container. Dilutions of the test serum are added. After a suitable time for reaction, excess antibody is removed by washing. Fluorescein-tagged antiglobulin (IgG) (prepared in the same animal species from which the nonlabeled serum was taken) is added. Fluorescence indicates whether or not there has been a reaction between antigen and the test serum. The indirect procedure is more sensitive than the direct as more sites for combination are available. Commercial kits are available to test for antibodies to many microbial diseases.

Radioimmunassay (RIA)

In this assay to detect antibodies, radiolabeled antibody competes with the patient's nonlabeled antibody (serum) for binding sites on a known amount of antigen. The radioactivity of the antigen-antibody complex is measured and compared with a control test containing no antibody bound to antigen. The greater the amount of radioactivity, reflective of the binding of the radiolabeled antibody to the antigen-antibody complexes, the higher is the antibody titer. This procedure can be reversed in order to detect antigen.

Because of the expense of equipment needed for RIA, and the hazards of radioactive reagents, ELISA systems, chemiluminescence and immunofluorescence assays are preferred.

Radioallergosorbent Test (RAST)

This procedure is used in the diagnosis of allergies. It is a radioimmunoassay (RIA) used to measure the antigen-specific IgE; the ligand is a labeled anti-IgE antibody. The method is similar to RIA except that the antigen (allergen) is covalently linked to a cellulose disc instead of being noncovalently bound to the RIA plate. The presence of much more allergen on the disc makes possible the binding of small quantities of IgE present in the patient's serum and thus a high sensitivity.

Western Blot Immunoassay (Immunoblotting)

This procedure, outlined in figure 16.5, is used to detect protein antigens. The proteins are separated using SDS-PAGE (sodium dodecyl sulfate-polyacrylamide gel electrophoresis), then transferred electrophoretically to a nitrocellulose membrane (see fig. 16.5). Specific antibodies if present will bind to their corresponding antigenic band(s). To the bands of antigen bound to the nitrocellulose is added the antibody (e.g., the patient's serum) followed by a labeled anti-immunoglobulin (human). The detection system used to read the test will depend upon the label that was used.

The pattern of antibodies revealed can be used to determine if a patient is infected with a particular microorganism. This procedure is useful in dealing with microorganisms that elicit numerous cross-reacting antibodies. For example, this technique is used to verify positive ELISA results when a patient is suspected of having Lyme disease.

Immunogold Labeling

This is an antibody-based procedure, which is used with the electron microscope, to identify microorganisms and other structures in various samples. The technique has been particularly useful in diagnostic microbiology.

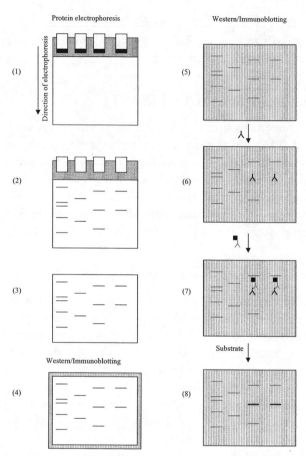

Figure 16.5. SDS-PAGE and Western/immunoblotting technique. (1) Samples are loaded into a SDS-polyacrylamide gel and subjected to electrophoresis. (2) Electrophoresis separates the protein fragments of an antigen based upon size. (3) The stacking (upper) portion of the gel is removed. (4) The gel is placed on a sheet of nitrocellulose and the proteins from the gel are transferred onto the nitrocellulose either electrophoretically or by capillary action. (5) the gel is then placed in blocking solution (typically bovine serum albumin or milk) to prevent nonspecific antibody binding to the nitrocellulose. (6) The membrane is then incubated with antibody, which binds specifically to the antigen. (7) The membrane is then incubated with enzyme-conjugated antibody (e.g., antihuman IgG). (8) The substrate for the enzyme is then added and allows for visualization of the antigen fragments to which the antibody binds.

This technique is carried out as follows: Antibodies are conjugated to gold beads of a particular size, for example, 10 nm (nanometers). Sections prepared for electron microscopy are blocked with a nonspecific protein and placed in a solution containing the antibody-gold conjugate. After incubation and extensive washing, the sections are examined with the electron microscope. Where antigen is present, it is surrounded by the gold beads which appear as round, dark spots as the electron beam is not able to penetrate the dense metal.

The procedure is also used in an immunohistologic technique in which tissue sections are stained with gold-labeled antibody. In a positive test the gold particles surround the target, such as microorganisms, and show up with the electron microscope as black dots.

Monoclonal Antibody

This is a single type of antibody, produced by a hybridoma cell line and directed against an antigenic determinant (epitope). The hybridoma cell line was formed by the fusion of a lymphocyte cell and a myeloma cell (from a plasma cell cancer). The procedure for obtaining a monoclonal antibody is outlined in figure 16.6.

Monoclonal antibodies have many uses in research and when labeled they are especially useful in the detection of pathogenic microorganisms.

Mixed Leukocyte Reaction

This technique is used for determining tissue matching for transplantation procedures. Leukocytes are obtained from both the donor and the recipient. These are then cultured together for several days. If reactive T cells are present, they will initiate T cell proliferation. After several days, ^{3}H- thymidine is added to the culture medium. Due to the massive amount of cell proliferation in a mismatching event, a great deal of ^{3}H-thymidine will be incorporated into the DNA of cells. This response will equate to a high amount of radioactivity as measured by a scintillation counter. However, if the cells are a good match, there is little T cell proliferation and little ^{3}H-thymidine incorporation, resulting in very low amounts of reactivity (see fig. 16.7).

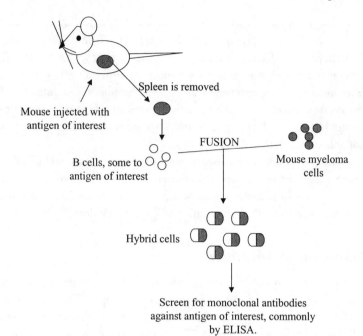

Figure 16.6. Production of monoclonal antibodies

FACS (Fluorescent Activated Cell Sorter)

This procedure allows for subsets of cells from mixed lymphocytes to be determined in a cell sample and allows for sorting so that one can examine a specific subpopulation of cells. In this technique, cells are collected and mixed with fluorescently labeled monoclonal antibodies to different cell markers. Typically, only one or two markers are used at a time. For example, if one wishes to determine the amount of CD4+ cells in a mixture (most probably predominantly Th cells), a monoclonal anti-CD4 antibody with a fluorescent dye attached to it would be used. After incubation, the cells are washed to remove excess, unbound antibody. The sample is then placed in a fluorescence-activated cell sorter (FACS), which sorts the cells into groups based upon the fluorescence present. This technique allows one to determine the types of cells present or percentages of cells expressing a particular cell surface marker. This technique is typically used in experimental situations.

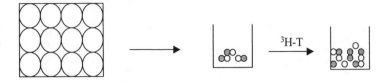

Microtiter plate

Figure 16.7. Mixed lymphocyte reaction. Donor (gray) and recipient (white) cells are mixed together in individual wells in a microtiter plate. Tritiated thymidine (^{3}H-T) is added to the culture media. If there is a reaction of the donor to the recipient or recipient to donor lymphocytes, the cells are stimulated to proliferate. DNA synthesis is used as the measure of cell proliferation, measured by the incorporation of the ^{3}H-T into the cells.

GLOSSARY

Acute and convalescent sera—sera collected at the acute phase of an infectious disease and when the patient is convalescing. If the titer of antibodies is appreciably higher in the latter serum compared with the acute serum it is considered evidence that a particular infection has been sustained.

Antiglobulin—antibody to a particular immunoglobulin, for example, IgG.

Fluorescein—a yellow dye that is used to tag or label compounds including antigens of microorganisms. This dye and related ones are visible under ultraviolet or other light sources including lasers.

CHAPTER 17

Human Immunodeficiency Virus (HIV) Infection and Acquired Immune Deficiency Syndrome (AIDS)

The occurrence of human immunodeficiency virus (HIV) infection leading to AIDS represents the most widespread, important and destructive infectious disease epidemic of recent years. A chapter is devoted to the disease because of its great significance and also because it illustrates a number of important immunological principles.

Before discussing the immunology of HIV infection and AIDS, it is helpful to have some general knowledge of the actual disease.

GENERAL

What we now call AIDS (acquired immunodeficiency syndrome) was first recognized clinically in 1981. Initially cases involved homosexual men and intravenous drug users. Later the disease was seen in individuals receiving blood transfusions, children of mothers injecting drugs, and bisexual men.

Prior to the discovery of HIV, the diagnosis of AIDS was based on the clinical finding of opportunistic infections such as pneumonia due to the widespread commensal protozoan *Pneumocystis carinii* and/or the presence of a rare skin cancer, Kaposi's **sarcoma**. As mentioned below other opportunistic infectious agents may also be involved. Opportunistic infections are caused by microorganisms to which normal individuals are generally resistant. This includes microorganisms that many of us carry as part of our normal flora and fauna. However, when the immune system is compromised by HIV infection or certain drug therapies, these organisms are able to cause disease.

One of two RNA viruses cause HIV. The first, HIV-1, was recognized and identified in 1984. HIV-1 is the causal agent in the United States and Europe. Since that time, many HIV-1 variants have been identified. HIV-2 was later identified as the agent of the disease in West Africa. These are genetically closely related retroviruses of the lentivirus family. The main features of the HIV-1 are illustrated schematically in figure 17.1.

HIV is found in semen and vaginal secretions and is spread by sexual contact, by the shared needles of drug users, and via placental transfer. Before blood was routinely tested for the virus, tainted transfusion blood was the source of many HIV infections.

Principal Opportunistic Infectious Agents in AIDS

The Centers for Disease Control (CDC) recognizes twenty-four different opportunistic infections as occurring as the result of HIV infection. The most commonly observed opportunistic infections are the following:

Toxoplasmosis. Toxoplasma gondii protozoan may infect various tissues including those of the central nervous system (CNS), and particularly the CNS of infants.

Pneumocystis carinii. A protozoan found frequently in the normal lung; cause of a serious pneumonia.

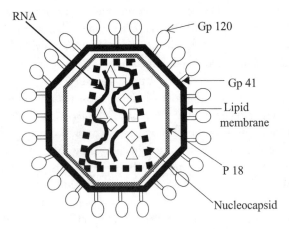

Figure 17.1. Schematic of HIV-1

Candida albicans. A yeastlike fungus that causes vaginitis and "thrush" (an infection of the oral cavity); it may become systemic and life threatening.

Histoplasma capsulatum. A soilborne fungus that is the cause of a systemic infection that can be fatal if not effectively treated.

Mycobacterium tuberculosis. A bacterium; tuberculosis was rare until HIV infections became widespread. The tubercle organism encountered in AIDS has been particularly virulent causing serious disease.

Mycobacterium avium complex. Bacteria that cause recurring fevers, digestive disturbances, serious weight loss, and general malaise.

Herpes simplex, types I and II. A virus, ordinarily the cause of minor infections; in AIDS patients, infections may be serious and massive.

Cytomegalovirus. Can cause pneumonia, infections of the brain and liver, and eye infections that can lead to blindness.

Cancers Associated with AIDS

Kaposi's sarcoma is the most common; it is a slow-growing tumor of the skin that can spread. B-cell **lymphoma,** caused by the widespread Epstein-Barr virus, is generalized and aggressive. Other cancers occur less commonly.

Neurological Disorders Associated with AIDS

These disorders are collectively called AIDS dementia complex. One cause is infection of the glial cells of the brain by HIV. It is thought that disturbances arising from infected T cells and macrophages in the brain may also be involved.

Stages of HIV Infection Leading to AIDS

The different stages of HIV/AIDS (as defined by the Centers for Disease Control) and their correlation with decreases in the number of CD4 T cells, the target cells of HIV, are presented in table 17.1.

THE VIRUS AND PATHOGENESIS

To understand the immunology of AIDS resulting from infection by HIV, it is necessary to examine the virus itself. As illustrated in figure 17.1, the

Table 17.1 Stages in the Progression to AIDS

Stages	Number of CD4 T cells per mm^3 of blood	Secondary infections
Before HIV infection	1,000	None
I. Acute illness; serum conversion. Symptoms in several days to several months; flulike symptoms; sero-conversion.	1,000	None
II. Chronic asymptomatic infection. Can be as long as 10 years.	800–500	Tuberculosis
III. Lymphadenopathy. Swollen and tender lymph nodes; flulike symptoms may recur; lasts several months.	500–200	Candida, Herpes I
IV. ARC* and AIDS. Disease now called AIDS; time until death usually 1 to 2 years.	200 and below	Opportunistic infections (see text), AIDS-related tumors, neurological disorders.

*AIDS-related-complex

virus has some essential features that account for its pathogenicity. As shown in figure 17.2, the HIV RNA contains nine genes. The *gag, pol,* and *env* are the major genes associated with the virus. The *env* gene encodes for the envelope genes *gp 120* and *gp 41*. The *gag* gene encodes for the core proteins, the matrix protein, and the nucleocapsid. The *pol* gene encodes for the enzymes reverse transcriptase, integrase, and protease.

The virus possesses a viral envelope, which contains many spikes consisting of the glycoprotein 120 kilodalton (gp 120) and gp 41 (fig. 17.1). It is the gp 120 that interacts with the CD4 molecule present on some cells (fig. 17.3, #2). Current research indicates that other receptor

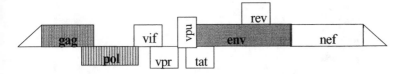

Figure 17.2. Schematic diagram of the gene arrangement of HIV-1. The genome is approximately 9200 nucleotides in length. At either end are terminal repeats, which are sequences that aid in viral DNA integration into the infected cell's chromosomes.

interactions in addition to that of the CD4-gp 120 are required for the virus to gain entry to the cell. The CC-CK5 receptor (CK-5) is an example of a **chemokine** receptor found on the surface of T cells and macrophages. The CK-5 is thought to interact with the gp 41 envelope protein. Apparently, the CD4 and CK-5 proteins interact to allow HIV to fuse with the cell and release its RNA. The CK-5 receptor must be expressed on the surface of the target cell, in addition to CD4, for successful viral entry into the cell.

After entering the target cell, other components of the virus come into play (fig. 17.3, #3). The two identical strands of viral RNA then enter the cytoplasm of the target cell. Along with the RNA, the viral enzymes reverse transcriptase, protease, ribonuclease (RNase H), and integrase also enter the cytoplasm (fig. 17.3, #4). The enzyme reverse transcriptase immediately begins the process of transcribing the viral RNA into DNA (Fig. 17.3, #5). Once this has occurred, and the DNA becomes double stranded, the original viral RNA is quickly degraded by another viral enzyme, RNase H (fig. 17.3, #6). The viral DNA then penetrates the nuclear envelope and enters the nucleus where the viral enzyme integrase is responsible for integrating the viral DNA into the cell's genome (fig. 17.3, #7). If the cell is not activated to respond to a particular antigen, the integrated virus remains latent within the host genome. From a clinical aspect, this initial infection is responsible for the "flulike" symptoms reported by HIV-infected individuals within a few weeks following infection. The asymptomatic stage following these flulike symptoms, which can last for years, is the result of the cell not being activated. However, some of these individuals have impaired Th function as a result of viral DNA integration.

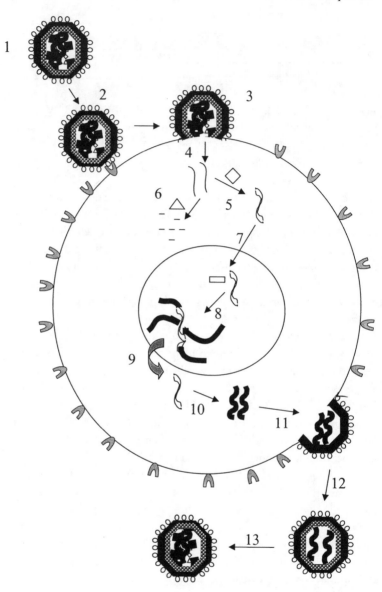

Figure 17.3. HIV life cycle. See accompanying text for description of each of the steps.

With cellular activation, the overt symptoms of AIDS appear. Activation of the cell stimulates a variety of viral genes from the previously latent integrated viral DNA. The transcription of the viral genome is mediated by the production of three accessory viral genes: *tat,* which speeds up transcription of the integrated DNA; *nef,* which modifies the infected cell to make it more suitable for producing HIV viral particles; and *rev,* which promotes expression of the HIV late structural genes (fig. 17.3, #9–11). Additional accessory genes *vif* and *vpr* (*vpu* in HIV-2) encode proteins that are involved in generating increased levels of HIV virions with consequent infectivity and pathologic effects. The cell essentially becomes a viral assembly factory. Transcription and translation of the HIV viral components, as well as the RNA genome, spontaneously assemble into viral particles and begin budding off from the infected cell (fig. 17.3, #12). The enzyme protease is involved in cleaving the translational products into their individual proteins, as they are synthesized in one long transcriptional piece from each of the three major genes (fig. 17.3, #12). The completely assembled virus is then available to infect another CD4 cell (fig. 17.3, #13).

Targets for the treatment of AIDS based upon this life cycle include reverse transcriptase, integrase, tat gene product, and protease.

IMMUNOLOGY

HIV binds to the CD4 molecule of helper T cells and then gains entry to these cells. Macrophages/monocytes and B lymphocytes are also infected. Proliferation of the virus may end with destruction of the CD4+ cells. When the CD4+ cells are sufficiently reduced in number, individuals become susceptible to the opportunistic infections and AIDS develops (table 17.1). The period from initial HIV infection to the development of AIDS is usually about ten years. The majority of cases, although improved with treatment, terminate fatally. Depletion of the CD4+ lymphocytes results in a decrease of cytokines, such as interleukin-2 and gamma interferon, resulting in monocyte/macrophage dysfunction. The progression of AIDS is reflected in the number of viable CD4 cells (see table 17.1).

HIV infects, but does not kill, **dendritic cells** and macrophages and thus they serve as sources of infectious virus in the infected individual. Macrophages transport virus throughout the body including the nervous system. The wasting syndrome seen in AIDS is attributed to compounds produced by infected macrophages. These cytokines, which are found to be in very high levels, cause the body to alter its metabolism. This results in patients needing more caloric intake in order to maintain their current body weight.

A controversial treatment for the wasting syndrome is the use of the drug thalidomide. Thalidomide was used in the 1950s to control the symptoms of "morning sickness" in pregnant women and tragically resulted in severe birth defects in children. It has been found to be useful for increasing the body weight in patients exhibiting wasting syndrome. However, a disadvantage of thalidomide treatment is that it appears to increase the number of HIV virus particles.

Infection of B cells may result in a hypergammaglobulinemia. The loss of B cells and CD4+ lymphocytes result in a poor antibody response to new antigens. Antibody-mediated cell cytotoxicity and lymphocytotoxic antibody may be responsible for the destruction of some HIV-infected lymphocytes. As the disease progresses both kinds of antibody are associated with decreases in CD4+ cells. This disturbance affects both cellular and antibody-mediated responses. The defect in cell-mediated response is predominant in adults, making them vulnerable to the intracellular infectious agents involved in Stage IV AIDS (see table 17.1). The lack of specific antibodies in children make them particularly susceptible to bacteremic infections due to *Haemophilus influenzae* and pneumococci.

VACCINATION

The development of an effective live attenuated vaccine, as is used to prevent many viral diseases, seems unlikely in the case of AIDS. The risk, although remote, of such a live vaccine causing AIDS, a highly fatal disease, is too great.

Stimulating the production of antibodies alone by a vaccine may not be effective, as antibodies are present in HIV-infected individuals. The surface antigen gp 120 that binds to CD4 is a highly conserved antigen and has been studied for its potential as a vaccine. The antigens p18 and p24 located within the virus are thought to be of no value as vaccines because antibodies to them would not be able to bind to intact virus (see fig. 17.1).

There are several HIV vaccines currently in different stages of development. In adults (over the age of twelve) a vaccine consisting of IL-12 is being tested to determine its efficacy in enhancing immunity in patients with HIV and *Mycobacterium avium* complex infection. For children (under age thirteen) with AIDS, an experimental antiviral compound known as 141W94 is coupled with an anti-reverse transcriptase inhibitor and used as an attempt to decrease viral load.

There are other potential vaccines currently being investigated for use in uninfected individuals to protect against HIV infection. However, these are all in the experimental stages of development.

DIAGNOSIS

An enzyme-linked immunoassay (EIA) is highly sensitive and able to detect more than 99 percent of infected individuals. Antigens used are the core protein p24 and the glycosylated envelope protein. The Western blot assay is used as a confirmatory test before a definitive diagnosis of HIV infection is made. The EIA is inexpensive and semiautomated; while the Western blot is able to detect antibody to all the viral proteins, but is labor intensive and expensive. Other confirmatory procedures used are a radioimmune precipitation assay and an immunofluorescence assay.

There is a period, from the time of infection to just before the first antibodies appear (seroconversion), when the HIV assays are negative. The core protein p24 circulates for several weeks before antibodies appear and it can be detected by an EIA using antibody for p24, although in practice the procedure would appear to have limited utility. During the period before seroconversion, virus can be isolated from cultured lymphocytes and a **PCR** procedure can be used to amplify proviral DNA from lymphocytes or RNA from plasma. Although this technology is available to detect the virus early in the progression of the disease, it would be limited to larger facilities.

TREATMENT

Azidothymidine (AZT) was the first drug approved for the treatment of AIDS. It acts by blocking the retrovirus enzyme, reverse transcriptase (RTC). It has extended the life span of patients although resistance to the drug has developed. A number of related drugs have been developed with a mode of action similar to AZT, but resistance has also developed toward them. AZT treatment is now known to be effective in blocking placental transfer of HIV to the fetus of the infected mother. In addition to AZT, other nucleoside reverse transcriptase inhibitors are didanosine, zalcitabine, statvudine, lamivudine, and abacavir.

A related class of drugs that works in a different manner is called the nonnucleoside reverse transcriptase inhibitors. Compounds of this group that are currently in use include nevirapine, delaviridine, and efavirenz.

The third class of drugs used in AIDS therapy target and inhibit the enzyme protease. The protease inhibitors currently approved for use in AIDS patients include saquinavir, indinavir, ritonavir, nelfinavir, and amprenavir.

Current drug treatments that are considered to be successful are the so-called drug cocktails. These consist of combinations of drugs with different modes of action: for example, an RTC inhibitor in combination with an inhibitor of the viral enzyme protease. By using this strategy, the potential for encountering a strain of HIV that is resistant to all three drugs simultaneously is very low. Another approach is the production of the protein gp 120, which binds to CD4 cells and thus blocks viral binding. Unfortunately, these approaches have not been very successful.

New drugs known as fusion inhibitors have been introduced recently that are designed to inhibit the fusion of the HIV with the plasma membrane and thus allow entry of the viral RNA and enzymes. These drugs, as well as integrase inhibiting drugs, are currently in various stages of clinical trials.

One of the most recent approaches to treatment involves antisense drugs. These are "mirror parts" of the viral RNA that disrupt the functioning of the viral RNA. One such drug is currently in the early phases of clinical investigation.

There has been considerable progress in the treatment of opportunistic infections resulting in improvement of the quality of life for AIDS patients.

IMMUNE RESTORATION

This is a current, although controversial, attempt to repair damage done to the immune system of HIV-infected individuals. One method of immune restoration is to remove some of an individual's immune cells, culture them *in vitro,* and infuse them back into the individual. Another method is to stimulate the production of more immune cells using cytokine therapy, especially IL-2, which stimulates the growth and proliferation of T cells. Gene therapy is also used to render bone marrow cells resistant to HIV infection.

Other aspects of immune restoration include (1) early treatment with antiviral drugs and allowing the immune system to repair damage with time; and (2) stimulating an HIV-specific immune response by immunizing HIV-positive individuals with killed HIV vaccines. These are thought to stimulate an immune response to HIV prior to activation and aggressive viral production, thus halting progression of the disease.

GLOSSARY

Bacteremic infection—an infection in which bacteria are present in the blood.

Chemokine—a family of cytokines whose functions are chemotaxis and the activation of other properties for a variety of cell types of the immune system.

Dendritic cell—an antigen-presenting cell that is present in the spleen, lymph nodes, and at low levels in blood. They are very active in stimulating T cells and are essential for primary immune responses.

Lymphoma—a malignant tumor of lymphoid tissue.

PCR (polymerase chain reaction)—a technique for producing many copies of a DNA segment without cloning.

Sarcoma—a malignant neoplasm of mesodermal origin, that is, of connective tissue, bone, cartilage, or striated (voluntary) muscle.

Cumulative Glossary

This glossary contains all of the definitions included in the glossaries at the end of chapters.

acquired immunity—immunity that develops as a result of a specific response to an organism or antigenic substance.

acute and convalescent sera—sera collected at the acute phase of an infectious disease and when the patient is convalescing. If the titer of antibodies is appreciably higher in the latter serum compared with the acute serum, it is considered evidence that a particular infection has been sustained.

adaptive immunity—see **acquired immunity.**

adenosine deaminase—an enzyme that is abundant in the thymus and in normal lymphocytes. Its deficiency results in the disruption of adenosine metabolism and the accumulation of toxic metabolites in the precursors of lymphocytes.

adjuvant—a substance, frequently given with the antigen, that non-specifically enhances the immune response to that antigen.

agranulocytosis—a condition in which there is a pathological fall in circulating neutrophils due to depression of myelopoiesis. There is a lowered resistance to bacterial infection along with, frequently, a severe pharyngitis, and if not reversed, septicemia, meningitis, or other conditions may ensue.

allele—an alternative form of a gene situated at corresponding sites on a homologous chromosome.

allelic exclusion—the situation observed with regard to gene rearrangement in germline T and B cells, where one chromosome is rearranged and prevents the use of the information on the second chromosome of the pair.

allergen—an antigen capable of eliciting an IgE antibody response. The latter antibody is sometimes referred to as reaginic antibody.

allogeneic—see **allograft.**

allograft—a graft between individuals of the same species who are sufficiently different that they interact antigenically, that is, they are allogeneic.

anamnestic response—the secondary, particularly strong immune response, which takes place some time after the initial or primary immune response.

anaphylatoxins—a group of substances that act as mediators of inflammation. They are produced during the activation of the complement cascade.

anergy—the phenomenon whereby lymphocytes that have been primed by an antigen fail to respond on second contact with the antigen.

antibody—a glycoprotein, one of five classes of immunoglobulins, produced by plasma cells. It has the capacity to recognize and bind to foreign molecules such as those on the surface of pathogenic organisms.

antigen—a substance, usually external to the body but occasionally within the body, which the immune system recognizes as foreign or nonself. When thus recognized it elicits a specific antibody that reacts with it.

antigenic determinant—see **epitope.**

antigen presenting cell—a cell capable of breaking down protein antigens and eventually displaying the peptide fragments complexed with the major histocompatibility complex on the surface of the cell. Once on the cell surface, the antigen peptide fragment plus major histocompatibility complex are available to interact with specific T cells. Some examples of antigen presenting cells include macrophages, Langerhans cells, dendritic cells, and B cells.

antiglobulin—an antibody against a particular antibody class or immunoglobulin, such as IgG. It is used in serological procedures to detect the presence of globulin.

antiserum—a serum containing antibodies; sometimes referred to as an immune serum.

antitoxin—an antibody that is active against a toxin.

apoptosis—a form of programmed cell death characterized by the fragmentation of nuclear DNA.

atopy—the clinical manifestation of type I hypersensitivity reactions, such as asthma, rhinitis, and eczema.

autoimmunity—the production of antibody-mediated or cell-mediated immunity to the constituents of the body's own tissues.

autologous—derived from self.

autosomal recessive defect—a recessive genetic defect involving a chromosome not involved in sex determination.

autosome—a chromosome other than a sex chromosome.

bacteremic infection—an infection in which bacteria are present in the blood.

BCG—Bacille (Bacillus) Calmette-Guérin. Named for French researchers, this is an attenuated strain of *Mycobacterium tuberculosis* used as a vaccine for the prevention of tuberculosis.

blastomycosis—a potentially serious fungal infection of humans and some animals caused by the soilborne fungus *Blastomyces dermatiditis.*

cAMP—derivative of ATP that occurs widely in animal cells as an intermediary messenger in many biochemical reactions induced by hormones.

catabolism—the breakdown of inorganic or organic compounds, usually leading to the production of energy.

CD44—a type I transmembrane protein that is found in many tissues and on many cell types.

cerebellar ataxia—the inability to coordinate muscular movements.

chemiluminescence—the emission of light (photons) from a chemical reaction. The chemiluminescent substrate luminol is used with horseradish peroxidase and the luminescent (light) response is detected with photographic film.

chemokine—a family of cytokines whose functions are chemotaxis and the activation of other properties for a variety of cell types of the immune system.

chemotaxin—a chemical stimulus responsible for the movement of cells.

chemotaxis—movement of cells to a particular location such as an inflammatory site, under the influence of chemotaxins.

cloacal opening—the common chamber of avian species into which the intestine and urinary tracts open and discharge wastes.

commensalism—a parasitic state in which the organism lives in or upon its host without causing disease. The organism benefits from the relationship but the host may or may not.

complement—a complex of serum proteins that act with and without specific antibody in a number of processes including inflammation, the activation of phagocytosis, and lytic action on cell membranes.

conjugate—a reagent formed by coupling covalently two molecules such as fluorescein and an antibody molecule. Conjugates are used widely in diagnostic laboratories to identify specific antigens of pathogenic microorganisms.

convertase—an enzyme that changes a substrate from one form to another.

Crohn's disease—a disease mainly affecting the small intestine (regional ileitis) and characterized by cramps, diarrhea, local abscesses, weight loss, and inappetence. The cause is not known.

cyclosporin A—an immunosuppressive compound derived from a soil fungus, that is used to suppress graft rejection.

cytokines—soluble molecules that mediate interactions between cells.

cytotoxic—having the ability to kill cells.

dalton—a unit of mass used to express masses of atoms, molecules, and nuclear particles. It is equal to one-twelfth of the weight of the carbon 12 atom; it is also called atomic mass unit.

defensins—small cationic, bactericidal peptides generated by peptides.

dendritic cells—antigen-presenting cells that are present in the spleen, lymph nodes, and at low levels in blood. They are very active in stimulating T cells and are essential for primary immune responses.

de novo—afresh, anew, from scratch.

dimer—a compound formed by the union of two molecules or two radicals of a simpler compound.

disulfide bonds—these form as a protein folds to its native conformation. They function to stabilize the protein's three-dimensional structure.

doubling dilutions—a procedure for preparing serial dilutions. The dilution of reagents in each tube, well, or other container is double that of the previous one, that is, 1 in 2, 1 in 4, 1 in 8, 1 in 16, and so on. Dilutions are made with pipettes.

emigration—movement between endothelial cells and into tissue at the site of injury.

endotoxin—a complex lipopolysaccharide (LPS) molecule composing the cell wall of some bacteria.

enteropathy—a disease of the intestinal tract.

epithelioid cells—these large cells are found in palisades in granulomas. They are thought to be derived from macrophages.

epitope—an antigenic determinant. It stimulates an immune response and binds specifically to antibody.

exocytosis—the release of secretory products from cell vesicles.

Fas (CD95)—a type 1 transmembrane protein of the TNFR (tumor necrosis factor receptor) superfamily. It is expressed on many cell types including those of the myeloid cell series.

fluorescein—a yellow dye that is used to tag or label compounds including antigens of microorganisms. This dye and related ones are visible under ultraviolet or other light sources including lasers.

Golgi apparatus—an assembly of vesicles and folded membranes in cells that receives, further modifies, and transports secretory products such as hormones and enzymes.

Goodpasture's syndrome—this disease is due to a proliferative glomerulonephritis and the principal symptom is the coughing of blood (hemoptysis).

gram-positive, gram-negative—the Gram stain is widely used in the identification of bacteria. With this procedure some bacteria remain colored (gram-positive) and some are decolorized (gram-negative). Gram-positive and gram-negative bacteria differ in the structure and composition of the cell wall.

granuloma—an aggregation and proliferation of macrophages and lymphocytes in response to certain chronic infections and foreign bodies. The immune response involved is a delayed-type hypersensitivity. The macrophages when compressed are called epithelioid cells. The granuloma is a roughly round lesion of variable size made up of mainly epithelioid cells that has at its center necrosis, the causal agent and various cells.

hairy cell leukemia—a leukemia characterized by an enlarged spleen and an abundance of large mononuclear cells whose irregular surface projections give a flagellated or hairy appearance.

helminths—parasitic worms including nematodes (roundworms), trematodes (flukes or flatworms), and cestodes (tapeworms).

heparin—this compound, which occurs in the liver and lungs, is used to prolong the clotting time of blood.

heterodimer—a protein consisting of two polypeptide subunits. Each of the subunits is different in its amino acid structure.

hexamer—a polymer formed of six molecules of a monomer.

histoplasmosis—a potentially serious fungal infection of humans and some animals caused by the soilborne fungus *Histoplasma capsulatum*.

Hodgkin's disease—a lymphoma (neoplasm) characterized by the progressive enlargement of the liver, spleen, and lymph nodes. Normal lymphoid cells are replaced by neoplastic, multinucleate giant cells.

homopolymer—a polymer consisting of identical monomer (one that can undergoes polymerization) units.

hyaluronidase—this enzyme breaks down and thus lowers the viscosity of hyaluronic acid, a mucopolysaccharide that is an important constituent of tissues.

hypoplasia—a condition whereby an organ, tissue, or part thereof is arrested in its development.

immune sera—sera that contain protective antibodies.

immunological tolerance—a state of nonreactivity to antigen that ordinarily would induce humoral or cell-mediated immunity. Immune tolerance may be produced in adults from administration of large or small amounts of antigen or contact with antigen in fetal or early postnatal life.

immunorepellents—bacterial immunotoxins that are specifically toxic for leukocytes.

interleukins (IL)—a number of low-molecular-weight proteins produced by lymphocytes and monocytes that mainly function in the regulation of the immune system.

isotype—when applied to immunoglobulins, isotype describes the immunoglobulin class, immunoglobulin subclass, light chain type and subtype. It can also apply to the variable region.

kinase—an enzyme that catalyzes the transfer of phosphate groups from ADP or ATP to a substrate.

leptospirosis—a disease affecting humans and domestic animals that is caused by spirochetes of the genus *Leptospira*.

leukemia—an acute or chronic neoplasm characterized by an abnormal increase in the number of leukocytes. It is classified according to the kind of leukocyte most prominently involved.

leukotrienes—a group of metabolites of arachidonic acid that have a number of pharmacological effects. They may be released from mast cells, leukocytes, and platelets.

levamisole—a drug used as an anthelmintic (mainly against nematodes) and also in cancer therapy.

ligand—refers to molecules that bind to cells or other molecules.

lipopolysaccharides—these have a lipid linked to a polysaccharide and are also referred to as endotoxins. They are derived from gram-negative bacteria and have various functions including adjuvancy (enhances the immune response) and acting as a mitogen for B cells.

lipoteichoic acid—teichoic acids intimately associated with lipid. They are found in gram-positive bacteria.

lymphoma—a malignant tumor of lymphoid tissue.

lymphopenia—a reduced lymphocyte count.

lymphosarcoma—a malignant lymphoma (a tumor involving lymphoid tissue) with a tendency to metastasize.

lysozyme—an enzyme found in saliva, tears, and nasal secretions that mainly lyse gram-positive bacteria.

major histocompatibility complex (MHC)—the collection of genes coding for the self-marking proteins or major histocompatibility antigens. These antigens occur on the surface of all the body's cells and serve to identify them as belonging to the body and not foreign. Some MHC antigens appear on the surface of cells of the immune system. The human MHC region is known as the HLA (human leukocyte antigen) region and is located on chromosome 6.

margination—sticking to the endothelium.

microthrombi—small thrombi. A thrombus is an aggregation of blood elements that can cause vascular obstruction at the point of its formation.

monoclonal antibody—a single type of antibody, produced by a hybridoma cell line and directed against an antigenic determinant (epitope). The hybridoma cell line is formed by the fusion of a lymphocyte cell and a myeloma cell (from a plasma cell cancer).

multinucleated giant cell—large cells that are formed by the fusion of macrophages. They are most prominent in granulomas associated with foreign bodies.

multiple myeloma—a neoplasm of the bone marrow characterized by the presence of numerous myelomas in various bones. The cells involved in myelomas may be any one of the bone marrow cells.

N-formylated (bacterial peptide)—it has a formyl group on the nitrogen of a particular amino acid, typically the first methionine in a protein.

nonapeptide—a peptide with nine amino acids.

opsonization—the promotion of phagocytosis by specific antibody in conjunction with complement.

peptide—a compound consisting of two or several amino acids.

phenotype—the expressed character of an organism.

plasma cells—mature B cells that have been stimulated by the combination of specific antigen and cytokines (intercellular mediators) to produce antibodies.

platelet—a small nonnucleated disc found in mammalian blood that is important in blood clotting.

polymerase chain reaction (PCR)—a technique for producing many copies of a DNA segment without cloning.

premunition—a state of protective immunity that occurs when small numbers of pathogenic organisms, especially bloodborne protozoans, persist within the host.

prostaglandins—a number of hormonelike compounds that have a variety of functions as inflammatory mediators.

protease—an enzyme that hydrolyzes or breaks down protein.

pseudopodium—the temporary protrusion or retractile process of the protoplasm of a cell.

receptor—a cell surface molecule to which particular proteins or peptides bind.

reticuloendothelial system—a term used to designate large mononuclear phagocytes associated with reticular tissues and endothelium. It includes both blood monocytes and fixed macrophages such as the Kupffer cells of the liver and those lining the sinuses of the spleen and lymph nodes. Additional cells with little or no phagocytic activity, such as dendritic cells, are also included. The term "RES" is now seldom used. It has been replaced by the more accurate term, the "mononuclear phagocyte system."

sarcoidosis—a disease of unknown cause characterized by nodules mainly in the lymph nodes, skin, lungs, and bones.

sarcoma—a malignant neoplasm of mesodermal origin, that is, of connective tissue, bone, cartilage, or striated muscle.

schistosome—blood nematodes or flukes that cause schistosomiasis; a severe disease occurring mainly in Africa, Asia, and South America.

signal transducton—this is similar to signal hypothesis and is the accepted explanation for the entry of light and heavy chains of immunoglobulins into the endoplasmic reticulum. This ensures the secretion from the cell of assembled immunoglobulin molecules.

teichoic acids—a class of strongly acidic polymers that occur in the cell walls, capsules, and membranes of all gram-positive bacteria.

thrombocytopenia—a decrease in the normal number of blood platelets.

T lymphocytes—cells of the immune system that mature in the thymus and are involved in the cell-mediated immune response.

transmembrane—across or through the cell membrane.

tuberculin—A protein extract obtained from the cells of *Mycobacterium tuberculosis.*

vasoactive amines—compounds produced by various cells that act on endothelium (lining cells of blood vessels) and smooth muscle of the local vasculature.

vasodilation—widening of the lumen of blood vessels resulting in increased blood supply.

viremia—the presence of virus in the host's blood.

xenogeneic cells—this term refers to grafted tissue derived from a species different from the recipient.

X-linked (sex-linked)—in sex-linked genetic disorders the mutant gene is located on the X chromosome. In females the gene is recessive when the partner gene is normal. As the male has only one X chromosome, he will be affected if the X chromosome carries the mutant gene.

zoonotic—diseases that are capable of being transmitted from animals to humans.

zymosan—an insoluble, mostly polysaccharide fraction of yeast cell walls.

Index